THE HEALTH OF
THE COMMONWEALTH

In the Pennsylvania Historical Association's *Pennsylvania History Series*,

edited by BEVERLY C. TOMEK and ALLEN DIETERICH-WARD

RECENT TITLES IN THIS SERIES:

Judith Ridner, *A Varied People: The Scots Irish of Early Pennsylvania*

Roger D. Simon, *Philadelphia: A Brief History*,
revised and updated edition

Judith Ann Giesberg, *Keystone State in Crisis:
The Civil War in Pennsylvania*

G. Terry Madonna, *Pivotal Pennsylvania: Presidential Politics
from FDR to the Twenty-First Century*

Karen Guenther, *Sports in Pennsylvania*

Marion Winifred Roydhouse, *Women of Industry and Reform:
Shaping the History of Pennsylvania, 1865–1940*

Daniel K. Richter, *Native Americans' Pennsylvania*

JAMES E. HIGGINS

THE HEALTH OF
THE COMMONWEALTH

A BRIEF HISTORY OF MEDICINE, PUBLIC HEALTH,

AND DISEASE IN PENNSYLVANIA

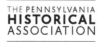

THE PENNSYLVANIA
HISTORICAL
ASSOCIATION

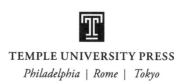

TEMPLE UNIVERSITY PRESS
Philadelphia | Rome | Tokyo

TEMPLE UNIVERSITY PRESS
Philadelphia, Pennsylvania 19122
tupress.temple.edu

Published by Temple University Press in partnership with The Pennsylvania Historical
  Association

Library of Congress Cataloging-in-Publication Data

Names: Higgins, James E., 1977– author.
Title: The health of the Commonwealth : a brief history of medicine, public health, and
  disease in Pennsylvania / James E. Higgins.
Other titles: Pennsylvania history studies.
Description: Philadelphia : Temple University Press, 2020. | Series: Pennsylvania history
  series | Includes index. | Summary: "This book is a history of medicine and public health
  in Pennsylvania from the colonial era through the present day, with coverage of medical
  advances, disease outbreaks, alternative therapies, and other topics that both link the
  state to broader national and international narratives and emphasize its residents' unique
  contributions"—Provided by publisher.
Identifiers: LCCN 2019056760 (print) | LCCN 2019056761 (ebook) |
  ISBN 9781932304695 (paperback) | ISBN 9781932304336 (pdf)
Subjects: LCSH: Medicine—Pennsylvania—Philadelphia—History. | Public health—
  Pennsylvania—Philadelphia—History. | Epidemics—Pennsylvania—Philadelphia—
  History.
Classification: LCC R313 .H54 2020 (print) | LCC R313 (ebook) |
  DDC 362.109748/11—dc23
LC record available at https://lccn.loc.gov/2019056760
LC ebook record available at https://lccn.loc.gov/2019056761

Printed in the United States of America

9 8 7 6 5 4 3 2 1

For my amazing wife, Sue

CONTENTS

Editors' Foreword, by Allen Dieterich-Ward
and Beverly C. Tomek   ix

Acknowledgments   xi

Introduction: *Of Plagues and Pennsylvanians*   1

1 Medical Frontiers, 1681–1804   5

2 Debating Disease, 1805–1865   25

3 Triumph of the Allopaths, 1866–1905   44

4 Triumphs and Tribulations of Public Health, 1906–1945   68

5 Promise and Peril of Private Medicine, 1946–2017   87

   Conclusion: *Keeping the Commonwealth Healthy*   104

   Afterword: *COVID-19 in Pennsylvania*   106

Notes   109

Index   121

EDITORS' FOREWORD

ON BEHALF OF THE MEMBERS and officers of the Pennsylvania Historical Association (PHA), we are pleased to present the third book in the newly redesigned *Pennsylvania History Series* (*PHS*). As part of the PHA's mission to advocate and advance knowledge about the history and culture of Pennsylvania and the mid-Atlantic region, the *PHS* remains dedicated to providing timely, relevant, and high-quality scholarship in a compact and accessible form. Volumes in the series are produced by scholars engaged in the teaching of Pennsylvania history for use in the classroom and broader public history settings. As we passed the seventieth anniversary of our first publication in 1948, a new partnership forged with Temple University Press now provides the series with the expertise, resources, and support of a respected academic publisher.

Dr. James Higgins's scholarship on medicine and public health first came to our attention when his 2014 essay on B. Franklin Royer won the PHA's Philip S. Klein prize for best article published in the journal *Pennsylvania History*. We were delighted when Jim accepted our subsequent invitation to submit a proposal for a volume on the topic for the *PHS*. While by no means comprehensive, the result is the first book of its kind to provide an overview of medicine and public health in the state from the earliest colonial era through the challenges of the present day. The book also provides close readings of specific medical advances, disease outbreaks, alternative therapies, and other topics that both link the commonwealth to broader national and international narratives and emphasize its residents' unique contributions to this history. In the end, *The Health of the Commonwealth* certainly demonstrates its central premise, noted in the Introduction, that "the history of medicine in Pennsylvania is no less vital to understanding the state's past than is its political or industrial history."

We thank Jim for providing such a timely, thoughtful, and engaging book that is sure to serve as a touchstone for future research on the topic. Thanks also go to our peer reviewers for excellent feedback that significantly improved an already strong initial draft. Our work as series editors is made possible by the support and guidance of the *PHS* editorial board as well as the financial commitment and leadership of the PHA Council. We are grateful for our friends at Temple University Press, who once again have worked their magic by turning a raw manuscript and some image files into the polished book that you now hold in your hands. Finally, we recognize Karen Guenther, who retired as PHA business secretary in 2019 as this book headed into press. For more than a decade, Karen played a vital role in shepherding the series through multiple editors, filling orders, and promoting our books at annual meetings.

—ALLEN DIETERICH-WARD, Shippensburg University

—BEVERLY C. TOMEK, University of Houston, Victoria

ACKNOWLEDGMENTS

Writing a book is never a solitary affair. I thank the Pennsylvania Historical Association (PHA) for selecting me to write *The Health of the Commonwealth* and especially my patient and tireless PHA editors, Beverly Tomek and Allen Dieterich-Ward. Their encouragement and prodding ensured that the project moved forward and bettered it in innumerable ways. The staff at Temple University Press could not have been kinder or more professional, and every burden they placed on themselves lessened my labor. The archivists at the Historical Society of Pennsylvania, the Pennsylvania State Archives, the Catholic Historical Research Center of the Archdiocese of Philadelphia, the Bradford Regional Medical Center, the Lehigh County Historical Society, the historical library of the College of Physicians of Philadelphia, and the Lehigh Valley Health Network provided invaluable service throughout the research preparation for the book. Professor Roger Simon, my mentor at Lehigh University and beyond, remains a constant presence in developing my research. Finally, the patience and good humor of my wife, Sue, who traipsed through archives, cemeteries, historical sites, and countless traffic jams, made my work possible.

THE HEALTH OF
THE COMMONWEALTH

INTRODUCTION

Of Plagues and Pennsylvanians

URING THE SUMMER OF 1793, ships from the Caribbean brought an unwelcome but all too frequent visitor to Philadelphia—the yellow fever virus. The virus had caused repeated, though relatively limited, outbreaks in the city since at least the early 1700s, but the epidemic of 1793 was different. Not confined to the docks or even the city, the virus spread along the watersheds of the Delaware, Schuylkill, and Susquehanna Rivers, sickening and killing victims a hundred miles from the city's harbor. Confusion about the origins of the sickness, how to prevent it, and treatments swirled among Philadelphia's medical community and civil authorities. In the end, cold autumn weather ended the outbreak, though some doctors insisted that their efforts brought the epidemic to a close. Almost two centuries later, in 1976, another mysterious disease emerged in Philadelphia. Most of the victims were in some way connected to a single hotel and a convention it hosted. Reaction by the medical community in the city and state was swift; victims who died were autopsied, tissues collected, and tests run to identify the cause. Within months of the first case, scientists identified a bacterium responsible for causing an infection the press dubbed Legionnaires' disease. With the pathogen identified, authorities mandated effective preventive measures while clinicians devised treatment regimens.

The history of public health and medicine in Pennsylvania links the state to a larger narrative of health and disease throughout the United States and the world. The great plagues of yellow fever, cholera, influenza, and AIDS that swept America and the globe also killed hundreds of thousands of the commonwealth's citizens. In its fight against disease, humanity has constantly sought to formulate effective preventive measures and medicines, and in this effort the achievements of Pennsylvania's universities, hospitals, and scientists influenced the well-being of people far beyond its borders. It is hoped that readers will come to realize the central role Pennsylvania played in humanity's understanding of, and progress against, disease. To be sure, the state's history of medicine has not been uniformly successful; urbanization boosted death rates for decades, as it did in every industrialized nation in the nineteenth century, while diet-associated diabetes, cardiovascular disease, and certain forms of cancer, to say nothing of AIDS, gun violence, and drug abuse, continue to take the lives of the state's citizens. *The Health of the Commonwealth*, then, is an evolving narrative whose contours stretch back to the earliest days of the colony and into a future filled with unforeseen challenges.

Yet Pennsylvania's medical history is not an absolute template for other American states because its history is unique. Not only did Pennsylvania begin as a colony long before colonials came to dominate the rest of British North America, but its founding as an experiment in religious tolerance under a benevolent proprietorship marked Pennsylvania as different from other colonies. Its largest town, Philadelphia, grew into the greatest city and port in the colonies. As industrialization transformed the world's socioeconomic conditions, laborers drew from its ground the coal and iron that remade the bucolic state into the nation's industrial powerhouse. By the turn of the twentieth century, Philadelphia and Pittsburgh offered different pictures of American cities; the former was the most ethnically homogenous in the nation, the latter the most diverse in terms of ethnic and racial makeup. When other states either had no medical schools or, even worse, possessed only diploma mills whose classrooms produced little more than laymen who masqueraded as physicians, Pennsylvania counted a half dozen medical programs, two of which ranked among the best in the nation.

Historians have not ignored the medical history of the state, but no definitive statewide history of medicine exists. To be sure, scholars found the medical histories of Philadelphia and Pittsburgh attractive subjects to research. One of the earliest monographs was J. H. Powell's 1949 work, *Bring Out Your Dead: The Great Plague of Yellow Fever in Philadelphia in 1793*, still a standard in the field seven decades after its publication. Industrialized Philadelphia proved an even more fertile field for explication, with Sam Alewitz's *Filthy Dirty: A Social History of Unsanitary Philadelphia in the Late Nineteenth Century* an outstanding overview of the environmental degradation present in every quarter of the city. Michael P. McCarty's *Typhoid and the Politics of Public Health in Nineteenth-Century Philadelphia* reminds readers that simplistic explanations that reduce environmental decay and disease to by-products of the age ignore the political decisions that helped propagate such conditions even after technology existed to reduce deaths from waterborne diseases.

The stunningly poor conditions in Pittsburgh, meanwhile, produced a slew of environmental and medical histories. This field of study in Pittsburgh is dominated by the works of Roy Lubove, whose two-volume study, *Twentieth-Century Pittsburgh*, is a touchstone in the field, while Joel Tarr's two comprehensive works, *Devastation and Renewal* and *The Search for the Ultimate Sink*, are both imaginative retellings of Pittsburgh's environment as well as incisive analyses of pollution and pollution abatement in the city. Between Pennsylvania's two great cities lay the interior of the state, largely rural and dotted with small villages and towns. Though the scholarship on this area, home to millions of the state's residents by the twentieth century, remains thin, Karol K. Weaver's article "'She Knew All the Old Remedies': Medical Caregiving and Neighborhood Women of the Anthracite Coal Region of Pennsylvania" and her book *Medical Caregiving and Identity in Pennsylvania's Anthracite Region, 1880–2000* offer insights into the important role of women and medical care in the small towns and tiny patches of the state's eastern coal fields.

THE HEALTH OF THE COMMONWEALTH rests on the premise that the history of medicine in Pennsylvania is no less vital to understanding the state's past than is its political or industrial history. Students of Pennsylvania's past often overlook the impact that disease, and efforts to combat disease, exerted on the state's history. This is a grave mistake. Perhaps the explanation for medicine's absence from the public's understanding of Pennsylvania's history is found in the influence that great political, military, and industrial moments in Pennsylvania's history exert over the imagination. When people remember the seminal moments in Pennsylvania's history, most recall the events of 1775 and 1776 that culminated in the Declaration of Independence, the protracted hardship of Valley Forge, and the bloodbath at Gettysburg. Great trends in Pennsylvania, for instance the dominance of the coal, iron, and steel industries, and the postindustrial collapse of each of those economic engines, are also familiar. With the exception of large epidemics, the subtle course of disease and healing that influences the lives of all people often eludes even the keen observer; most people know intuitively that throughout much of Pennsylvania's past people lived without benefit of modern medicine, that soldiers wounded on the state's battlefields faced grim prospects for recovery, and that sanitation was primitive. These realities are accepted as simply the conditions of life in the past, conditions that seemed to have straightened themselves out in a rather linear progression with the steady march of time and science.

Of course, we do not accept that industrial methods, weapons technology, political change, or any other facet of human endeavor were simply destined to progress. Instead, we acknowledge that important decisions and actions, both planned and accidental, taken by people, some well known and others obscure or unknown, defined the course and progress of, for instance, the iron and steel industry. The same is true of health and medicine in the commonwealth. At times, Pennsylvania reformers and scientists changed the course of medical history for the better, perhaps most notably in the case of the first polio vaccine, which was developed at the University of Pittsburgh. A delay of only a year in the delivery of the vaccine would have condemned thousands more children to their graves or mechanical breathers for the rest of their lives. Fifty years earlier in the same city, water purification was delayed for a decade because of political fighting over the distribution of graft-laden contracts connected to the construction of the purification system. The delay was responsible for the deaths of thousands of people who need not have died from waterborne illness. The history of medicine is not solely a technocratic history but rather a techno-social history that requires not just an understanding of science but also a recognition that technology must be implemented, and people—politicians, physicians, and the public—have the final say over what technology is adapted, for whom, and at what pace.

A fair narrative of the state's medical past encompasses not only the sort of scientific medicine that most people associate with "real" medicine but also the Native American medicine, premodern European folk medicine, and unconventional medical practices that competed with allopathic medicine.[1] Furthermore, constructing the medical history of Pennsylvania demands great emphasis on the role of public health, especially the great achievements in sanitation and water purification that have saved untold numbers of lives, and on the role of public medicine—for example, the building of the state's immense tuberculosis sanitaria and the great Philadelphia public hospital, Philadelphia General. Both public health and public medicine reduced morbidity and mortality in the state long before effective treatments were developed for most diseases. While not a seamless narrative, *The Health of the Commonwealth*, I hope, conveys the many strands of disease, medicine, and public health thought and practice throughout Pennsylvania's historical eras coherently and with due attention paid to the overall historical context.

1

MEDICAL FRONTIERS, 1681–1804

PENNSYLVANIA REFLECTED THE PRESENCE of diseases and healing practices from throughout the Atlantic littoral. The rapid imprint of myriad healing traditions alongside the arrival of a slew of infectious diseases from Europe, Africa, and Asia largely resulted from the commerce and people attracted to Philadelphia. Laid along the west bank of the Delaware River, Philadelphia squatted on swampy bottomland cut by numerous creeks and one significant river, the Schuylkill. Surrounded by marsh, the city was humid and hot throughout summer, with winters damp and sometimes bitterly cold. Beyond the reaches of the town, elevation increased and hills emerged as the land rose to meet the foothills of the Appalachian Mountains, whose sharp ridges and infrequent gaps formed the first great natural impediment to European settlement. Between the Delaware River and the mountains lay the forests from which colonists hewed their settlements, even as disease and war ravaged the indigenous peoples.

Health and Disease on the Farm and Frontier

Native Americans confronted disease and devised their own system of medicine in Pennsylvania long before the first European set foot on the west bank of the Delaware River. For thousands of years, people inhabited the mountains and valleys of what became Pennsylvania, free from the innumerable infectious diseases that stalked humanity in Europe, Africa, and Asia. This is not to suggest that the pre-European inhabitants of Pennsylvania lived in a world devoid of disease. On the contrary, indigenous communities were subject to traumatic injuries, infected wounds, and infectious diseases such as Lyme disease and hantavirus. Precolonial peoples devised ways to bind fractures and close wounds, as well as poultices and herbal remedies to stave off infection and reduce fever. Depicting pre-European Pennsylvania as a sort of Eden-like paradise unfairly minimizes the dangers people faced and the ingenuity of their medicine.

Disease, more than warfare and privation, was most responsible for the catastrophic loss of life among the Susquehannock and Lenni Lenape east of the Allegheny Mountains. The decline began in the 1600s as contact with Europeans, and their germs, increased. The Susquehannock claimed lands along the Susquehanna River and the Appalachian Mountains just to the west of the Blue Ridge. During the 1660s and 1670s the tribe's population declined precipitously, likely because of smallpox, with survivors absorbed into neighboring groups.[1] The largest Native American group, the Lenni Lenape, claimed the land east of the Blue Ridge, from New York to Maryland and Delaware. Like the Susquehannock, the Lenni Lenape faced decimation, with villages in closest contact with colonists affected by disease earlier than those in the interior of eastern Pennsylvania.

That infectious disease wreaked such havoc on native populations in Pennsylvania was the result of two factors. The first was simple deprivation—of food, shelter, peace—in the face of colonial expansion. Though the history of Pennsylvania's relations with the Lenni Lenape in the decades following the colony's founding emphasized the relative lack of violence, penetration of settlers into the colony's interior spread disease and undermined the stability of village and tribal life.[2] The second and most important factor was the vulnerability of all indigenous people in the Americas to the diseases of the Eastern Hemisphere. Because of a variety of interrelated causes, the immune systems of indigenous peoples throughout the Americas were ill-equipped to resist European, African, and Asian pathogens. The disease, war, and privation experienced by native populations throughout the Americas culminated in the most catastrophic loss of life in history, and despite the positive narrative of European–Native American relations in Pennsylvania with which most are familiar, Pennsylvania's native population faced the same near extinction that cultures throughout the Americas suffered when confronted by colonists and their microbes. As the Native American population declined in the eastern third of Pennsylvania, colonists replaced them, with homesteads and crossroads growing into villages and towns.[3]

The enormous loss of life among Pennsylvania's Native Americans in just the century following the colony's founding limited the experience Europeans and colonials had with Native American medicine. Nevertheless, observers noted the expertise with which the Lenni Lenape cared for wounds and extracted foreign bodies, including musket balls, with a skill not matched by the most proficient colonial surgeons. Treatments for skin problems, including burns and boils, were effective, and success was claimed with the bite of the copperhead and rattlesnake.[4] Unfortunately, Native Americans' unfamiliarity with Eurasian and African diseases put them at a terrible disadvantage not only immunologically but therapeutically. Unused to treating epidemic infectious disease, Native Americans in Pennsylvania were judged poor nurses by colonials, their sick "left to die in the woods," while even close relatives would bring the sick only "a little food and drink."[5] Unfair characterizations by Europeans and colonials aside, the Lenni Lenape possessed an outstanding knowledge of medicinal plants that they used to soothe the symptoms of infectious disease, including those brought by Europeans. Also of note was the Lenni Lenape's habit of coupling herbs and other treatments while calling on the supernatural, a habit not dissimilar to the folk medicine that eventually took root in Pennsylvania.

Reliable figures concerning the extent of infectious disease among Europeans who lived beyond Philadelphia remain difficult to ascertain, but generalities may be made. It is certain that isolated communities and farms suffered the same sicknesses that stalked colonists in Philadelphia and throughout Europe. The major difference between Philadelphia and rural communities was not the variety of diseases each suffered, rather it was the frequency with which disease visited; towns and farming families might not see a particular disease for years. Unfortunately, when a pathogen did alight in a more remote community after a long absence, most or all of a town's nonimmune population fell ill. In such cases, children constituted an outsized portion of the vulnerable population, and outbreaks sickened and killed the young disproportionately. Indeed, epidemics in the small hamlets that dotted Pennsylvania east of the Appalachians could carry away young children from every household in just a few weeks, leaving survivors reeling.

Medicine was first and foremost a family affair, an activity carried on overwhelmingly by women—mothers, wives, and daughters were the primary caregivers.[6] The scarcity of doctors of any sort in rural sections made the knowledge and expertise of women especially critical to the recovery of the ill and injured. Larger towns in the counties and towns outside Philadelphia, for instance Germantown, Reading, Lancaster, and Bethlehem, were home to a variety of "country doctors," many of whom had no formal medical schooling and relied only on their observation of other country doctors for their medical training. Furthermore, no hospitals existed in rural Pennsylvania. When illness struck, caregivers—physician and lay—utilized what prepared medicines they had, as well as herbal preparations derived from medicinal plants. The flora utilized in Pennsylvania included species brought from Europe as well as those native to North America. Studies of rural healers during the colonial era, most of them women, highlight the nexus of European and Native American healing techniques, especially with regard to the search for medicinal plants in the colony that reproduced the effects of the Old World herbals with which healers and physicians were already familiar.[7]

The women on whom colonial Pennsylvanians relied to heal the sick in rural areas came in many forms: most were simply people whom others believed were adept at curing illness through herbs, poultices, and the like; some were elder women of a community whose lifelong experience with disease proved valuable to less experienced households. Midwives remain the best known and researched class of healer in the colonial world. Their presence was especially important among the farming folk of the colony, where even country doctors were few. Furthermore, the midwife's duties often went far beyond the birthing stool to include treating people of all ages and both sexes through illness, injury, and preparations for burial of the dead.[8] Midwives were often mischaracterized by contemporary physicians—with whom they increasingly competed—as incompetent and even dangerous to mothers and newborns because of a supposed lack of skill, as well as by historians, who often portrayed midwives as "cunning folk," a reference to old women in English villages whose lives provided a template for tales of witches in early modern Europe.

For many communities and isolated farms, however, the reality was much different; midwives offered the only skilled medical care beyond what a wife or mother could provide, and the expertise of an experienced midwife usually exceeded that of a rural doctor. Just like regular physicians, midwives and other informal healers sometimes used regular assistants as nurses and cultivated gardens filled with medicinal herbs, an especially important task in regions where the supply of medicines prepared in Europe or colonial cities was not usually available.[9] The ubiquitous colonial midwife and associated healers who relied on herbs and their own experience to heal were joined by another class of healer specific to Pennsylvania, a group reputed to harness the supernatural, along with herbs and other remedies, to effect healing.

The great wave of German immigrants who entered Pennsylvania in the early eighteenth century brought a strong tradition of healing based on Christian beliefs. The Pennsylvania Dutch, as Pennsylvania Germans were eventually called, blended their European folkways with Native American healing practices and the flora that grew in the region to develop a hybridized version of healing called "powwowing."[10] Powwowers utilized sacred symbols such as crosses, stones, and other items thought to have either healing properties or the ability to draw out curses—or hexes in the vernacular of the Pennsylvania Dutch. Powwowers did not generally claim the power to cure acute diseases such as cancer or sudden heart attack, though some practitioners insisted that powwow medicine could staunch heavy bleeding; rather they concentrated on minor ailments—tooth- and earaches, sleeplessness, and the like. The healing process demanded that both practitioner and patient believe in the power of powwow and Christ to relieve illness or banish hexes.

The rich tradition of such practices, as well as the centrality of women in the healing arts, may be distilled in the life of a woman who lived in the hills of Oley Valley, about fifty miles outside Philadelphia. Anna Maria Jung (Young), popularly known as Mountain Mary, was born about 1749 in Germany and, with her parents, immigrated to colonial Pennsylvania, probably Germantown, in the decade before the Revolutionary War.[11] Verifiable information about Mary is scant, and what exists has been intertwined with supposition and myth, but Mary, with her mother and two sisters, left Germantown after their father died, probably of disease, and perhaps as a result of the Battle of Germantown. They settled in District Township, now part of Pike Township, in Berks County. Mary's mother probably died by 1790, as the census listed only three women, likely Mary and her sisters, in what sources indicate was a rough-hewn log cabin.[12] Most importantly, the census listed Mary as the head of her household and, in a census enumeration that rarely listed title or occupation even for men, Mary was listed as "the Abbess." Interestingly, the census did not list a surname for Mary, as "the Abbess" took the place of a family name. Her will, written in 1813, included forty acres, several hundred dollars, two of the most prominent men in the county as beneficiaries or executors, and a desire to pass on her manuscripts and books to interested parties.[13] Her will, which identified her as never married though possessed of a modicum of wealth, marked Mary as different from most women.

A few months before her death in November 1819, two men journeyed to her farm and remarked on its order and her industry. Mary expounded in German about God and religious devotion, showed her interlocutors the graves of her family members, and then set out fruits and cheese on a table, all of them superior in quality and produced by her own hand. After her death, stories of her power as a healer spread throughout the county, especially in the region near the Oley Hills. The scholar cannot rely on heroic stories that, while compelling, cannot be verified. The census description of Mary as "the Abbess" seems to identify her as not only a religious person but

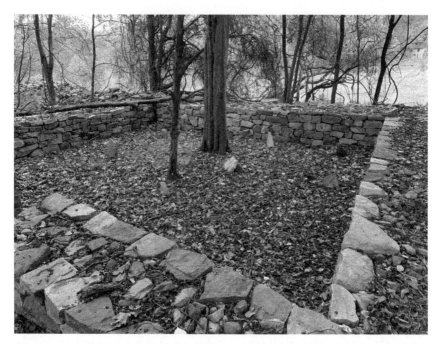

The private grave of Mountain Mary in Berks County, Pennsylvania. The other graves are likely siblings and her mother. (Courtesy of Sue Higgins.)

perhaps the leader of some sort of religious community, or at least a person locally recognized as uniquely spiritual and/or religious.[14] Use of the particularizing "the" in the census may even indicate that Mary's role as religious healer was a widely understood fact in the southeastern farmland of Berks County. The census data, as well as her will, also dispel the many myths that surround her. Anna Marie Jung was not some sort of reclusive Pennsylvania witch, as she is sometimes portrayed, who lived a solitary existence among her gardens and farm animals; she was a minor religious leader, was literate, and lived with close family.[15] Her status as a healer may be disputed by the scholar on the grounds that there is no written record to substantiate such a claim. However, Mary's status as a healer is congruent when one understands that the Pennsylvania Dutch accorded certain people the ability to harness the power of folk medicine and God to heal the afflicted.

Strictly speaking, Mountain Mary was not a powwower, though she is usually identified as such. Regardless of the specifics of her method of practice, Mountain Mary and healers like her utilized herbs, diet, incantations, and basic nursing to effect healing and ward off evil. Mary's homestead still exists off Mountain Mary Road, a few hundred yards from the top of a ridge.[16] The current owners of the property, which has long since reverted to forest, maintain two dairy cows in honor of Mary's prowess at producing fine cheese. The graves of Mary and her family, marked by simple head- and foot-stones, any inscription long since erased by the elements, remain behind a low stone wall near the trails Mary may have taken to care for the sick in her community; a monument not to a witch or hermit, but to an educated woman who harnessed faith and experience to ease suffering and comfort the dying, in the best tradition of Pennsylvania medicine.

Rural healers enjoyed good reputations in their communities. People's perception of healers as competent, even preferable to the country doctor, indicated a trust inspired by more than spiritual conviction or the necessities of frontier life. Instead, the Pennsylvania folk or community healer may have forged a better record of preserving life and reducing suffering than their physician counterparts, two key elements that encouraged faith among patients and their families. By eschewing or limiting the use of treatments like bleeding, purging, and vomiting, healers avoided aggravating a patient's illness. If one accepts that neither physicians nor healers could cure infectious disease, but rather that they supported the body's natural defenses against disease, it follows that healers who caused the least insult to the body managed to restore to health a higher percentage of their patients than those who weakened them. Furthermore, Pennsylvania Dutch healers inflicted less suffering on their patients than conventional medical responses. This last point, alone, may have been enough to convince many to trust in the powers of powwow and other modes of healing.

Life and Death in the Colonial City

Throughout its history, Philadelphia has been the population center and major entry point for European and African migrants, free, indentured, and enslaved, for Pennsylvania. By the American Revolution, it was the largest city in the colonies and one of the largest ports in the British Empire. Colonial Philadelphia boasted some of the finest churches, universities, and hospitals in North America, but the white-stockinged, powder-wigged city of popular imagination is more myth than fact. Philadelphia, by eighteenth-century colonial standards, was indeed a city. Like every city, Philadelphia possessed neither an understanding of microbes nor the technology to construct anything beyond rudimentary public health measures. The result was an indescribably filthy environment that contained a host of disease hazards.

So deleterious to health was life in Philadelphia that through the mid-eighteenth century the city grew only because of the migration of people to the city from Europe and the surrounding countryside.[17]

A typical street in eighteenth-century Philadelphia consisted of a mixture of mud, straw, and manure, to which every citizen added the contents of chamber pots, food scraps, and other waste.[18] Rain and spring's thaw turned the streets into tracks of clinging mud, through which cart wheels cut deep ruts. In the yards and lots behind homes and shops stood the outhouses and cesspits into which Philadelphians poured their bodily waste, kitchen refuse, and household debris. Cesspits leaked their contents into the ground from which citizens drew their drinking water. Food, never cold in summer, rotted quickly and was adulterated by sellers to mask spoilage or increase volume. Dairy items proved especially dangerous, particularly for children, who depended on milk for an outsized share of their nutritional needs. Thousands of animals were butchered in the city, the remains of the carcasses processed to produce items like leather, which entailed the production of a great deal of wastewater. To the stench of the tanneries were added the foul odors and billows of acrid steam and smoke from bone-boiling and fat-rendering establishments. Rodents and flies thrived in Philadelphia, as did pigs and stray dogs, both of which ran semi-wild in the streets and in the stables that housed the city's cows, horses, and mules. In addition to microbial threats, people faced danger from traumatic injuries delivered by kicking horses, careening carts, and the knives and gunshots used to settle arguments in taverns and alleys, all of which required surgical intervention without anesthesia and in conditions seemingly designed to promote sepsis.

Life expectancy in eighteenth-century Philadelphia was decades shorter than in the early twenty-first century. Many of the deaths occurred in those under age ten. Newborns faced a host of dangers, including injuries and infections received during labor. Children under five were sensitive to diarrheal illness, most prevalent during the summer months and commonly the result of drinking excrement-laden water and food. The term "summer diarrhea" referenced such illness and death among infants. Those that survived infancy faced an army of pathogens against which they possessed little immunity. By the eighteenth century, with Philadelphia's population at more than two thousand, the germs that caused scarlet fever, diphtheria, measles, and other childhood diseases were yearly occurrences and killed hundreds annually. Death rates increased even more when epidemics broke out.

Smallpox was, until yellow fever surpassed its ferocity, the most feared disease of colonial Philadelphia. Caused by a virus, smallpox spread via droplets of fluid from the nose, throat, and lungs. Smallpox could also spread via infected bedding and clothing, though the airborne route was more significant. Ten days after exposure to the virus, a victim's fever rose, body aches developed, and exhaustion sapped sufferers of their energy. Smallpox also frequently provoked nausea and vomiting that could last for days. After a few days of influenza-like illness, symptoms subsided and spots appeared in the mouth and throat. Within three days, the body was covered with bumps that filled with fluid that leaked for as long as two weeks before finally drying, crusting over, and falling off. The scars left people disfigured and often blind. The mortality rate for uncomplicated smallpox hovered around 30 percent, though more virulent forms of the disease, which accounted for only a small proportion of cases, killed in more than 90 percent of cases. In Philadelphia, smallpox cases occurred every year and epidemics ignited every few years. The size of the city's population allowed smallpox to establish itself as an endemic (ever-present) disease in Philadelphia earlier than any other community in British or French North America.[19]

Though smallpox was Philadelphia's greatest killer, the litany of sick and dead recorded by town gazettes and parish records was mostly owed to far less spectacular sicknesses. Measles, for instance, raced through a community with stunning speed, its infectiousness greater than any pathogen on earth. The moderate fever and mild rash of measles belied its power to kill, especially when one managed to evade it in youth and instead contracted it in adulthood, as bacterial pneumonia often followed a bout of measles. Scarlet fever, its red rash followed by desquamation—the loss of large patches of skin—preyed almost exclusively on children under ten years of age, with deadly effect in about 10 percent of cases. Another serious disease, diphtheria, occupied an increasingly prominent position in the mortality rolls of European cities and Philadelphia during the eighteenth century. Infection with diphtheria was hideous both for victims and, as was often the case, for parents who tended their children. After a few days of fever and sore throat, the toxin produced by the bacteria caused a leathery membrane to form and stretch across the tonsils and, in the most serious cases, across the pharynx. Victims of diphtheria often remained conscious while they slowly asphyxiated or collapsed from heart failure.

Despite the ravages inflicted on Pennsylvania and its most important city by disease, the colony did enjoy one advantage from an epidemiological perspective: a long, cold winter that killed tropical mosquitoes and thereby prevented such species from establishing a breeding population.[20] Tropical mosquitoes like *Aedes aegypti* held the power to transform exotic insect-vectored disease from periodic threats that arrived aboard ships, as was the case in Philadelphia, to the same sort of endemicity that plagued British possessions in the Caribbean, Georgia, and South Carolina. In Philadelphia, malaria constituted the most persistent mosquito-borne threat, and though malaria could be deadly, the strains most responsible for causing the disease in the city were the least serious forms with which Europeans were familiar.[21] When a ship from the Caribbean docked, however, it sometimes brought the *A. aegypti* mosquito and the *Plasmodium falciparum* parasite responsible for the most lethal form of malaria. The malaria caused by *P. falciparum* produced high fevers and wracked sufferers with a cycle of chills so acute that teeth might break from uncontrollable chattering. Common neurological symptoms included confusion and lethargy, as well as encephalitis. In some cases victims passed dark urine, which gave rise to one name for the disease, "black water fever," the result of kidneys that failed to remove damaged red blood cells from the body, which built up in the kidneys and caused renal failure.

In addition to malaria, Philadelphia imported cases of two other mosquito-borne diseases. The less serious of the two, dengue fever, spread from Asia as the result of European colonization. Dengue has a relatively low mortality rate in the twenty-first century, but in combination with malnutrition and other disorders already weakening a victim, dengue can kill. The first positive outbreak in the city occurred in 1780, the fierceness of its body pains unlike anything physicians had before encountered.[22] So awful was the pain associated with the fever that many referred to it as break-bone fever or bilious remitting fever for the vomiting it caused and the curious nature of the fever, which tended to relent during the day and peak in the morning and at night.[23] The worst of the tropical illnesses, yellow fever, caused terror at the rumor of its approach. The virus caused high fever and uncontrollable vomiting. Worse followed for about 15 percent of those infected when the virus entered its hemorrhagic phase, during which victims bled into the whites of their eyes, their gums leaked blood, and the stomach bled. People unfortunate enough to experience this manifestation of yellow fever vomited partially digested blood, which gave rise to its nickname, black vomit fever. Worse still, the virus could damage the liver, which caused jaundice, hence the moniker yellow fever. Yellow fever resulted in death in more than 30 percent of cases in which bloody vomiting and liver damage developed.

Infectious disease, which ended the lives of most colonials, had for thousands of years been blamed on a variety of causes unrelated to germs. Perhaps the most popular explanation blamed noxious gases that emanated from swamps and cesspools. The odor of rotting vegetable matter, manure piles, and abattoirs caused suspicion, too, as did exposure to night air. So widespread and strong was the connection between disease and repugnant scents that the term malaria is derived from the Italian words "mal" and "aria," or "bad air." Another common name for a specific illness, influenza, was derived from the Italian for "influence." The influence to which the term refers is that of the celestial bodies as well as weather, especially the cold, damp conditions of winter when cases of the common cold and influenza peaked. Even as people blamed poisoned air and planetary bodies for disease, the humoral system of medical thought, which emphasized the role of bodily fluids, and the correction of an imbalance of those fluids in treatment, profoundly influenced the thinking of colonial physicians.[24] Some colonial Pennsylvanians also believed in the power of the supernatural to cause illness. The means by which the supernatural sickened people differed across cultures, but God, the devil, curses, and witchcraft were all culprits for people trying to make sense of the seemingly inexplicable visitation of disease.

Inaccurate models of disease causation spawned ineffective treatments, many of which originated in antiquity and grew no more efficacious with the passage of time. As it was generally assumed that inappropriate quantities of blood, phlegm, and bile caused disease, logic dictated that drawing off excess fluid eased symptoms and cured disease. The most familiar such treatment was bleeding. Far from a straightforward opening of the veins of the forearms, bleeding might be done at any point on the body, and often at locations that corresponded to a patient's pain, with cuts along the legs, chest, back, and genitals. The quantity of blood removed from the patient could amount to several pints over the course of a couple of weeks of illness. Far from therapeutic, bloodletting weakened the victim and could hasten death. As the eighteenth century closed, bleeding declined in popularity in Pennsylvania. Along with bleeding, purging of the bowels and use of emetics to induce vomiting composed a virtual trinity of standard initial responses to sickness, regardless of symptoms.

Medical Capital

The medical market in Philadelphia ranked as the colonies' most sophisticated, yet the majority of people availed themselves of folk medicine, or what one historian referred to as "'old-wives' remedies, 'kitchen physic,' and downright magic and superstition" to effect cures, just like their country cousins.[25] Medicine was by no means an exclusively white colonial affair; African slaves who evinced a talent for the healing and surgical arts were also called on to tend the ill. For example, an announcement in a 1740 Philadelphia newspaper gave notice that a slave named Simon, who could "bleed and draw Teeth, pretending to be a great Doctor," ran away and was worth a three-pound reward.[26] Though Simon and his master lived in New Jersey, some slaves in

Philadelphia were undoubtedly known for their talent as healers. The employment of kitchen physic and healers of all sorts is decipherable when one considers that science, though it might explain the movement of planets and
produce navigational aids, had hardly begun to penetrate the world of disease
and offered few dependable cures. Many doctors, and those who advertised
themselves as doctors, completed no formal training and were no more
knowledgeable about medicine than any experienced community healer,
whether in Philadelphia or its hinterlands.

Scholars generally recognize that doctors were organized into three
groups in the eighteenth century: physicians, responsible for curing disease
through a variety of medicines, therapies, and diet regimens; surgeons, who,
less prestigious than physicians, amputated limbs, extracted teeth, and removed objects (for instance, bullets) from the body; and apothecaries. In
colonial Philadelphia, and throughout the colony, conditions required doctors to acquire expertise in all three areas.[27] Training for doctors varied, and
many learned their trade by reading texts and apprenticing, alone. One of the
city's most celebrated physicians, William Shippen, for instance, learned
through books and without benefit of a mentor.[28] Shippen built one of the
most prestigious practices in the city and counted numerous leading citizens
as patients and friends. By the middle of the eighteenth century, would-be
physicians increasingly began their medical education in the colony and
earned their medical degrees in England, especially the University of Edinburgh. Two of Philadelphia's most influential physicians, William Shippen
Jr. and Benjamin Rush, graduated from Edinburgh. It was no accident that
the first medical school in North America, opened by the University of Pennsylvania in 1765, used as its model the University of Edinburgh's school of
medicine. Two decades later, in 1787, Rush and other doctors founded the
College of the Physicians of Philadelphia, an intellectual and social group
dedicated to the furtherance of medical knowledge in the colony and mod-
eled after the Royal College of Physicians in London.[29]

Physicians possessed a wide array of therapeutics, most of them ineffective or dangerous to patients. At the onset of illness doctors often employed
calomel, a form of mercury, to loosen the bowels, and ipecac to provoke
vomiting. After the general treatments of bleeding, purging, and vomiting,
physicians moved to treat specific areas affected by sickness. For lung ailments such as pneumonia and pleurisy, doctors administered caustic plasters
on chest and back to raise a blister and thereby draw out the poison thought
to cause the illness. In addition to using it as a laxative, physicians employed
mercury for a number of ailments, most importantly syphilis and other diseases that manifested skin eruptions. The metal might also be spread as an

ointment on the skin or inhaled. Though mercury sometimes reduced and even eliminated syphilis in some cases, the side effects included tooth loss, sores in the mouth, uncontrollable salivation, neurological symptoms, and death. Another popular medication was opium, which was usually mixed with liquor and drunk. Opium reduced pain and suppressed cough, though colonials often used it for other symptoms regardless of efficacy. Physicians recognized the danger of overdose associated with opium use, especially when administered by physicians and laypeople unfamiliar with its effects. However, as opium amounted to the single most potent and reliable pain reliever available in the eighteenth century and much of the nineteenth century, its use continued unregulated for centuries.

The most effective prevention for a major disease was smallpox inoculation, which was brought to Europe from Turkey in the early eighteenth century. By about 1735, inoculation reached Philadelphia and, as in every community, ignited debate over its use. Those against inoculation believed its use endangered the community. Such fears were not without merit. Inoculation involved scraping and collecting dried scab from smallpox skin eruptions. After mixing the powdered scab with inert material, an inoculator cut or abraded the skin of a patient and deposited the mixture into the wound. What followed was usually a mild to moderate bout of smallpox with fewer complications, lower mortality, and quicker recovery than naturally acquired smallpox. Besides infection of the inoculation site, which could progress to blood poisoning or gangrene, a larger threat did, indeed, loom in the community from inoculation; as patients did develop smallpox, they shed virus from their throats and the pocks that appeared on their skin. Any member of the community who had not already acquired immunity to smallpox either through prior infection or inoculation risked infection from an inoculated person. If one was infected by an inoculated person, the course of disease would be the same as naturally acquired smallpox. Other naysayers believed that the manner and time of one's death were best left in God's hands. From this perspective, inoculation placed the power of life and death in the case of smallpox in the hands of humankind, an unnatural and ungodly state of affairs.

The best argument for inoculation, that it reduced mortality from the disease, became more plainly clear as the eighteenth century wore on. The most powerful voice in support of smallpox inoculation in the city was Benjamin Franklin. In 1736, a wave of smallpox washed over Philadelphia, and though inoculation was available, Franklin delayed inoculating his beloved son, six-year-old Francis, so that the boy might recover from a bout of diarrhea. The delay proved fatal and Francis succumbed to smallpox. Within a few years, Franklin used his press and his reputation to push for voluntary inoculation for all citizens of the city and its environs. By the middle of the 1770s, Franklin engaged himself in the task of raising funds specifically designated to facilitate inoculation of the poor, who usually suffered terribly during outbreaks because they could ill afford the fee physicians charged for inoculation.[30]

During the same period Franklin began to raise money to inoculate the poor, 1777–1778, George Washington undertook to inoculate all new enlistees in the Continental Army at Valley Forge. This was especially important as the last continent-wide epidemic of smallpox was raging, especially in the larger ports, with hundreds dying in Philadelphia alone. By the turn of the nineteenth century, an improved version of protection against smallpox, vaccination, utilized the much safer cowpox virus to provide cross immunity to smallpox with small chance of serious complications. The physician who claimed to have introduced the new procedure to Philadelphia, John Redman Coxe, claimed that of patients who availed themselves of vaccination "perhaps nineteen of twenty scarcely exhibit a perceptible indisposition," especially compared to the earlier practice of inoculation.[31]

Apart from infectious disease, even natural biological processes posed serious threats to one's life. Labor and delivery was the most dangerous period of a woman's life. One study suggested that women of childbearing age in Pennsylvania suffered a mortality rate that was 40 percent higher than men in the same age group.[32] Through the mid-eighteenth century, midwives dominated caregiving during labor and delivery in Philadelphia. The role of midwives was a long-standing practice in English medicine and reflected the tradition of women tending to their daughters and sisters. By the Revolutionary War, however, as European medicine began to refine obstetrics with new techniques and instruments, much of Philadelphia's gentry opted for the care of physicians during delivery.[33] In 1795, when the daughter of noted Philadelphia diarist Elizabeth Drinker suffered a difficult labor, a physician was called to assist a well-known midwife. According to Drinker, "a bad presentation [of the fetus] had taken place . . . which . . . call'd for his skill more perticularly [sic]."[34]

Dr. William Shippen Jr. was the catalyst for much of this change as he brought new methods from Europe and instructed midwives and physicians on best practices for delivery.[35] Though many women and their families were reticent about inviting a male into such an intimate and traditionally female experience, and the transition to male-dominated obstetrics took decades, the esteem with which Shippen and other male physicians were held by leading Philadelphia families, and their increasing power to regulate medicine, progressively undercut the power of midwives.[36] Whether birthed by midwife or physician, the mortality rate of infants under one year of age through the mid-eighteenth century routinely exceeded 20 percent.[37]

The late eighteenth century also marked an important change in family planning in Philadelphia and other areas of the United States. Evidence suggests that families, especially those in cities and towns east of the Appalachian Mountains, began to have fewer births. Reasons for the drop in offspring included the rising price of land and the increased disapproval with which middling citizens in urban areas viewed child labor. Furthermore, the labor of children was less important for urban middle-class families in Philadelphia and the large towns in eastern Pennsylvania. Market forces, including consumerism, also played a role as urban families diverted money to the consumption of an increasing array of manufactured goods. The increasing literacy of women of all socioeconomic strata also allowed for the quicker transmission of information about abortifacients and contraceptive methods. This knowledge was generally well understood by the era's midwives but might now be promulgated to a wider audience of women who could both read and had a desire to use the methods in a comprehensive manner during the course of their childbearing years. Literature that confirmed the value of the smaller family also reached women readers.[38]

The health of all Pennsylvanians, especially those in crowded Philadelphia, would have been made better by a cleaner environment and better responses to disease outbreaks. But, as in the case of medicine, public health efforts—quarantines, sanitary services, and similar efforts—suffered from the paucity of accurate scientific knowledge about the cause of disease. As a rule, public health was a reactive force throughout the eighteenth century. When a particularly violent epidemic struck, mayor, council, and prominent citizens created a temporary board of health. With the exception of smallpox and yellow fever, many outbreaks were described hazily in terms of "distempers," "malignant fevers," and similar names.

Regardless of the etiology of the disease, Philadelphia—and every city in the British Empire—employed the same set of procedures.[39] Since medical experts throughout the empire and in Philadelphia believed that "when filth is acted upon by a hot sun in a moist state it produces fever," authorities sought to cleanse the air on streets with high rates of sickness by burning smudge pots, the contents of which included brimstone (sulfur), gunpowder, and urine-soaked hay, all of which produced gray, acrid smoke.[40] Smudge pots were also ordered burned in the homes of the infected and the dead. Sometimes the belongings of the dead or sick, usually the poor, were incinerated. Rubbish was collected and street gutters cleaned. Manure piles, too, were abated. Homes with sick and dead occupants could face quarantine, though clergy and physicians might come and go. Air and street cleansings, ineffective though they were in mitigating disease, conveyed the sense that something was being done to reduce the threat. Isolation of sick families offered some protection, but quarantine was rare, and the passage of clergy and doctors offered a chance for pathogens to spread.

The first concerted efforts the colony took to arrest the spread of disease aimed to prevent the transfer of disease from ships docked at the port of Philadelphia. As early as 1700, colonial authorities ordered inspection and quarantine of suspected cases of disease among crew and passengers.[41] Though the first generation of port inspection in Philadelphia was ad hoc, it did provide the precedent for expansion of the colony's medical infrastructure. Twenty years later, Philadelphia strengthened the inspection regimen by appointing a port physician specifically charged with inspection of crew and passengers. By 1743, in part to remedy the quarantine's porous nature and keep diseased people and ships as far as practical from the growing city, Philadelphia purchased land on Fisher's Island in the Delaware River about a mile south of the city center.[42] Colonial authorities maintained a very modest quarantine station on the island for people removed from ships; isolation of suspected cases of communicable disease, not treatment, was the primary aim. Eighteenth-century medicine remained unable to diagnose asymptomatic cases of disease, so quarantine, unless an entire ship's company was isolated, allowed people who could spread infection, but had not begun to show symptoms themselves, to enter the city.

Institutional medical care for citizens began with the opening of the Friends Almshouse for indigent Quakers in 1713. Meant to house the poor and put them to work, the Friends Almshouse could not avoid taking in the sick and offering basic care, even if on a temporary basis. More crucial to the development of Philadelphia's healthcare infrastructure was the Philadelphia Almshouse, which opened in 1732.[43] Though not a formal hospital, the Philadelphia Almshouse nevertheless offered both outpatient and inpatient treatment in its infirmary. The medical services it offered, which were integral to its charter and operations, argue for its designation as the first hospital in the colony and, under this logic, the almshouse predated even Bellevue (1736) in New York City as the first hospital in British North America.

The other institution that contends for recognition as the colony's first hospital, Pennsylvania Hospital, was founded by a consortium of physicians and prominent Philadelphians, including Benjamin Franklin, in 1751. Certainly the first conventional hospital in the colony, it was supported in part by colonial funds as well as contributions by donors and patient fees. The proposal for the hospital set as its mission the treatment of the city's poor, including those too destitute to pay for services, though affluent members of colonial society utilized the hospital's services too. Importantly, Pennsylvania Hospital set itself to the task of caring for the insane, a group widely abused both on the streets and in clinical settings in the eighteenth century.[44] Insofar as the colonial assembly provided funds for both the Philadelphia Almshouse's infirmary and Pennsylvania Hospital, these institutions were the first vehicles through which Pennsylvania's government delivered public medicine. In 1786 Dr. Benjamin Rush founded North America's first outpatient clinic for the poor, the Philadelphia Dispensary, which further bolstered public health efforts designed to aid the poor while providing a wealth of opportunities for physicians to observe and treat a wide variety of infectious diseases and traumas.[45]

Yellow Fever and Its Aftermath

As the eighteenth century closed and a new century dawned, Philadelphia underwent a series of changes in its public health infrastructure and medical thought. The catalyst for such change arrived from outside Philadelphia, on a ship from the Caribbean. Yellow fever activity in the West Indies increased by the beginning of the 1790s, and it was only a matter of time before it reached Philadelphia. The outbreak began in 1793 during the sullen heat of July and continued until cool mid-October weather killed the mosquitos. The worst-hit areas lined the waterfront, where the ships that carried mosquitoes and infected refugees from the revolutionary war in Saint-Domingue concentrated.[46] By September the epidemic virtually shuttered the city as New York and other communities closed their ports and roads to Philadelphia commerce and citizens. In the city, corpses began to turn up in alleys, lots, and buildings, their families and friends having fled in terror. Many of the wealthier people of the city removed themselves from the threat by escaping to the towns that ringed the city. The flood of those fleeing the city spared some but also spread the illness to towns like Harrisburg and Easton, which recorded fevers of unclear etiology but likely yellow fever.[47] The 1793 outbreak of yellow fever remains the worst outbreak of infectious disease in American history, with at least 5,000 deaths, or 10 percent of the population of the nation's largest city, and hundreds of others dead but uncounted outside the city. In the early twenty-first century, a similar mortality rate would have left 150,000 dead in Philadelphia alone.

The city's response to the epidemic included the standard repertoire of smudge pots, burning of possessions thought to be contaminated by the sick and the dead, and exhortations about the reasons for the disease's appearance. Authorities seized a large home, Bush Hill, on the edge of the city for use as an emergency isolation and treatment center for the poor, while a small death house was erected along the Schuylkill River.[48] In one of the great moments of collective courage during an American epidemic, black citizens who remained in the city nursed sick whites and gathered and buried the dead left behind by white family members and friends. Though their services were desperately needed, some whites criticized black citizens for their supposed greed as some wished to be paid for their services.[49] It must be remembered that in this regard African Americans who tended the sick and buried the dying expected little more than the remuneration their white counterparts received. In the face of such criticism, two prominent leaders of the city's African American community, Richard Allen and Absalom Jones, wrote that black citizens felt "sensibly aggrieved by the censorious epithets of many, who did not render the least assistance in the time of necessity, yet are liberal of their censure of us."[50] Benjamin Rush, too, believed Philadelphia's African American community served with distinction. Rush observed that during the epidemic his servant Marcus, a black man, "put up powders, spreads blisters, and [gave] clysters equal to any apothecary in town."[51]

The most public dispute in the wake of the 1793 yellow fever epidemic consumed Philadelphia's physicians and centered on two critical areas: yellow fever's origins and its proper treatment. Benjamin Rush, the most famous Philadelphia doctor of his era, believed the fever arose from sources within the city. In the case of the 1793 epidemic, Rush traced the cause to piles of rotting coffee on the waterfront.[52] As for the spread of the disease from one person to another, Rush believed "there was no instance of this disease being contagious."[53] A growing chorus of physicians disagreed and believed the disease was brought to the city by ships, and that people passed the disease to others, though the exact mechanism for such transfer (what would be called contagion in a few decades) was unclear.[54] Neither Rush nor those who opposed his views were absolutely correct in the case of yellow fever: The disease was not contagious between people—a mosquito was necessary to transmit the disease, though the virus infected mosquitoes when they drew a blood meal from someone already infected with the virus. The disease was also not a result of filth in the city; rather, the virus was brought to the city from places where the virus, and mosquitoes capable of transmitting the virus, flourished.

Even more heated than the debate about the causes of the disease were arguments about effective treatment. Rush advocated a regimen of bleeding and bowel purging, which he claimed cured almost every one of his patients.[55] Other physicians decried such methods and instead insisted that treatment of symptoms—palliative care—offered better hope for recovery. So fierce did the arguments between the factions become that one editor of a city paper accused Rush of unintentionally killing his patients, an accusation that resulted in a $5,000 libel judgment against the editor.[56] The debate among the city's physicians reflected a larger impulse in medicine at the end of the eighteenth century that diminished the value and role of bleeding as a medical treatment, and later did the same for purging and vomiting, in favor of less arduous interventions.

As passionate as the debate in medical circles became, the changes yellow fever wrought in Philadelphia's public health infrastructure were even more immediate and far-reaching. The year after the epidemic, 1794, the city founded a board of health responsible for recommending safeguards against disease even during nonepidemic periods.[57] Put another way, the 1794 board of health was the city's first permanent board expressly purposed to prevent epidemics, not react to them. As such, the city granted the board a budget to support twenty-five inspectors, several physicians, and a few administrators. In 1801, the Philadelphia Lazaretto opened on Tinicum Island several miles downriver from the city for use as an inspection point and isolation station for sick passengers. By 1808, the board was charged with gathering statistics on deaths from smallpox and other important diseases.[58] Registering deaths, and the causes of deaths in the city, was a prerequisite for understanding which illnesses caused the most deaths and the sections of the city with the highest mortality rates. The board's statistics presaged the growing recognition throughout the nineteenth century that a basic understanding of births, deaths, and causes of death was the first step in building a public health apparatus that might not only respond to epidemics but prevent them.

Conclusion

The casual observer may be forgiven for believing that the first one hundred twenty-five years of Pennsylvania's medical and disease history recorded few improvements. The evidence for such conclusions is ample; besides inoculation, no breakthroughs in treatment or revelations about the cause of infectious disease occurred. This view unnecessarily limits the measure of the colony's efforts to fight disease. In Philadelphia, the groundwork for its modern medical and public health structures were laid, including its first school of medicine, hospitals, and public health boards. In the debate between physicians about the efficacy of inoculation, and the later debate about treatments for yellow fever, the city recorded its first public splits among physicians with respect to older forms of treatments and new methods that seemed to promise better results. In rural Pennsylvania, the Pennsylvania Dutch and other communities established new folkways of healing, including the pow-wow tradition, utilization of native medicinal plants, and incorporation of Native American knowledge. The eighteenth century, then, was perhaps most important not for the cures that emerged, but rather for the path it carved for the next generation of Pennsylvania healers.

2

DEBATING DISEASE, 1805–1865

I T MAY BE FAIRLY STATED that the yellow fever epidemic of 1793 marked the close of eighteenth-century medicine and public health in Philadelphia. In the aftermath of the epidemic, debate raged about proper medical treatment for victims, the origins of the fever, and the need for improvements to the city's public health infrastructure. Philadelphia, and to some degree Pennsylvania, began to emerge from its past as a colonial medical outpost and move into the future as an autonomous people free to fashion their own medicine within the context of a new nation. The period between the yellow fever outbreaks of the 1790s and the end of the Civil War was also the interval during which hospitals, university-trained physicians, and efforts to standardize the quality of medical care moved beyond the confines of Philadelphia and began to affect health and medicine across the state. New medical challenges, notably cholera, also emerged during the early decades of the nineteenth century and spurred new ways of framing disease and its prevention and treatment, and once again highlighted the link between Pennsylvania and the wider world of medicine and disease.

Cholera

If yellow fever was Philadelphia's eighteenth-century epidemic touchstone, then cholera was Pennsylvania's quintessential nineteenth-century disease. In 1832 the disease emerged in Pennsylvania at just the moment when the state was experiencing the first throes of industrialization coupled with urbanization. A new urban middle class began to coalesce in the cities and large towns, conscious of their status and desirous of avoiding shabby sections of their communities and the filth and disease that lurked in such areas. Increasing numbers of immigrants, especially the Roman Catholic Irish, crowded into the cities and towns of the state, their wretched poverty, religion, and accent making them despised.[1] The propensity of the Irish to carry typhus, a lethal disease caused by a bacteria carried by the body louse, a species of vermin especially prevalent in the fetid holds and filthy clothing of Irish immigrant ships and the people they carried, condemned the Irish to the ranks of disease carriers, a moniker often hung around immigrants.

Into Pennsylvania's crowded cities and growing towns arrived cholera, the most acute gastrointestinal disease to which humans are susceptible. Most people who contract cholera do so by drinking water contaminated with fecal matter from those already in the throes of the illness. Cholera strikes suddenly and leaves victims doubled over in pain and unable to control their vomiting and diarrhea, even if the first symptoms begin in public. The watery discharge is usually white in color, hence the name "rice water stool," and carries bits of mucus and tissue from the lining of the intestinal track. Gallons of fluid, along with much of the body's electrolyte supply, pour from the body in just a few hours. With the lack of supportive care for sufferers in nineteenth-century Pennsylvania, their excrement contaminated bedding and clothing and posed a danger to caretakers. Victims grew cold to the touch, and their skin developed an unmistakable blue hue, their eyes deeply sunk into the face. As severe dehydration and electrolyte loss took their toll, muscles cramped and spasmed uncontrollably, the kidneys failed, and the heart's rhythm grew erratic. Victims could go from full health to death in as little as five or six hours. Death rates in severe cases of cholera in the nineteenth century were high, and for every one death there existed many minor or moderate cases.

For centuries, the bacterium that caused cholera remained confined to the delta of the Ganges River on the Bay of Bengal in India. Beginning in 1817, European military conquest and trade spread the disease beyond the Ganges and the Bengal and into much of Asia, the Middle East, and Russia by the time the first pandemic subsided in 1824. The second pandemic commenced in 1827, and by July 1832 Philadelphia felt its effects. In response to cholera, doctors, both regular and irregular, healers, and public health officials employed every means of prevention and treatment known to the era. The city's authorities washed streets with torrents of water from the Schuylkill River, detained ships at the quarantine station, opened emergency hospitals to isolate the infected, fired smudge pots, burned the clothing of the dead, and encouraged an exchange of ideas about proper treatments for the disease. Physicians suggested that "drunkards, and the debauched of every class, have been among the chief sufferers" of cholera in Philadelphia, along with "the indigent inhabitants, of low, damp, and ill ventilated portions of the city."[2] The conclusions of the physicians who wrote such reports were supported by the presuppositions in the minds of middle-class and elite citizens about the morals of the immigrants and African Americans who lived under such conditions.

Despite the best efforts of city officials and medical practitioners, thousands of people suffered cholera's ghastly symptoms and roughly a thousand died through the autumn. Though Philadelphia's poor suffered disproportionately, the city's mortality rate was less than half that of New York. Unsurprisingly, Philadelphia's leaders credited their quick action for keeping the city's mortality rate low, but there were likely other explanations. For one, as crowded as Philadelphia's poorer neighborhoods may have been, New York was even more densely populated. Of even more importance, at least in terms of explaining the higher mortality rates in the poor areas of Philadelphia, was the fact that the city took much of its drinking water from the Fairmount Reservoir, which stored water from the Schuylkill River above Philadelphia, and distributed it to hydrants and homes. The first centralized water supply in the nation, the water stored in the reservoir was raw river water polluted by communities upstream, but not nearly as contaminated with cholera bacteria as the city's wells and pumps that pulled up groundwater contaminated by adjacent cesspits. The majority of the residential water connections were in the homes of the well-off, while the poor made do with fetid groundwater. When the discharge of cholera victims was dumped into outhouse holes, the bacteria leached into the water table and thence into pails, pitchers, and cups. The system by which human fecal bacteria made its way from cesspits into drinking water and back into people is sometimes termed a circular water supply.

The epidemic of cholera in 1832 in western Pennsylvania was a much more subdued affair than it was in Philadelphia and its environs. Though the towns and villages dotting the Monongahela, Allegheny, and Ohio River valleys saw cases hit within days of one another, and Pittsburgh recorded cases a few days before Philadelphia, the city of thirty-five thousand people failed to act as a focus for cholera's spread. The good fortune of the western communities did not result from extraordinary sanitary measures; rather it was likely the region's sparse population and decentralized system of wells, streams, rivers, and springs that proved more difficult for cholera bacteria to infect or contaminate. Deaths throughout the region were measured in the scores, not hundreds.[3]

The power of a cholera epidemic to kill numbers of people quickly and stoke terror in a community is best glimpsed in an episode from one of Pennsylvania's small workers' camps. During August 1832, cholera struck a crew of fifty-seven Irish railroad workers laboring to construct a section of the Philadelphia and Columbia Railroad about thirty miles outside Philadelphia.[4] All fifty-seven Irish immigrants died over the course of a few days and were buried adjacent to the railroad. Though it was long assumed that the laborers all died from cholera, archeological findings in the early twenty-first century indicate some may have been killed by gunshot and blunt force trauma. Researchers suspect that cholera killed most of the workers, while a combination of anti-Irish/anti-Catholic sentiment and the terror of cholera spreading to families near the worksite doomed the others.

Two other epidemics of cholera swept Pennsylvania in 1849 and 1866, and the years between epidemics rarely saw the state completely free of the disease. From a biomedical perspective, an outbreak in 1854 in the town of Lancaster provides a window into the changes occurring in medical thought with respect to disease causation, as well as the maturation of Pennsylvania medicine. When the Lancaster outbreak began in late summer, physicians from Philadelphia investigated the epidemic. It appeared clear to some of the investigators that the disease was brought to Lancaster from other places, for instance the town of Columbia, Pennsylvania, which experienced a violent outbreak of the disease mere weeks before the outbreak in Lancaster began, as well as Cleveland, Ohio, where members of a family in Lancaster journeyed to care for kin infected in that city's 1854 epidemic.[5] It was, concluded some of the Philadelphia physicians who studied Lancaster's travails, more likely that people infected others with cholera, rather than that the disease sprang spontaneously from rubbish in the streets or filth in the water.

At exactly the same time Lancaster faced cholera, August and September 1854, Dr. John Snow undertook the study of an outbreak in London and traced its spread to a single pump on Broad Street. When he convinced authorities to remove the pump handle, the epidemic petered out. Snow's methods—compiling and tracking cases and deaths, as well as interrogating accepted models of disease causation to gauge their accuracy—are recognized as major steps in epidemiology and in the transformation of thought regarding the cause and spread of infectious disease. Though bacteria were not yet implicated in cholera and other infectious diseases, the theory of contagion—that people could infect others with their illness—steadily gained ground against older models of disease causation and marked an important shift in thinking. Incredibly, a group of Philadelphia physicians, well trained by American standards of the era, completed the same sort of work using many of the same methods that Snow developed to unlock some of the epidemiological secrets of cholera. The gulf that separated the great epidemic of yellow fever in 1793 as well as the first great epidemic of cholera in 1832, both of which learned medical minds blamed on rotting waste, from the last gasp of cholera in Pennsylvania in the mid-1860s, attributed to spread from one person to another, witnessed a major shift in Pennsylvania medicine.

Antebellum Medicine

The greatest development in medical thought and practice during the early to mid-nineteenth century was the advent of the Paris School of Medicine.[6] The Paris School emerged from the large hospitals of Paris, especially the Hotel Dieu, which afforded physicians and medical students the opportunity to observe numerous diseases in a diverse patient population. The Paris School stressed collection of data about each patient and the patient's illness, including temperature, rash, pulse, social condition, and assorted other information. Clinicians collected information on patients during regular rounds, the concept of rounds or regular checks on patients itself a new innovation. The Paris School accelerated the obliteration of thousands of years' of medical "knowledge" throughout the nineteenth century. Especially important was the doubt the Paris School threw on the role of "distemper," or an imbalance of bodily fluids and energy, and associated other ancient notions of disease causation, in favor of explicating the cause of sickness and death through observation of individual patients and the findings of autopsies.[7] While an imbalance in a single patient might, at least according to the logic of premodern medicine, cause disease, epidemics seemed to suggest that thousands of people became simultaneously distempered at once, an explanation that became increasingly untenable. As a corollary, cholera epidemics initiated a reexamination of the miasma theory and sanitary practices, with Britain's Edwin Chadwick and his fellow sanitarians prominent in reinventing urban sanitation. The theory of contagion—that people could infect others with their disease by some unknown mechanism—began to replace miasma and allied theories of disease causation. Though the fruits of the Paris School and Chadwick's work trickled into Pennsylvania unevenly, the decades before the Civil War were nevertheless a dynamic period of growth in Pennsylvania medicine.

A critical figure in transferring the new knowledge and methods of the Parisian physicians to America was William W. Gerhard, a Philadelphia doctor.[8] Born in 1809, Gerhard earned his medical degree from the University of Pennsylvania in 1830 and began his studies in Paris the same year. Gerhard observed a number of outbreaks in Paris and was so taken by the innovation he witnessed among French doctors that he wrote American physician-students were unable to do anything useful beyond acting as "interpreters to the Parisian pathologists."[9] When he returned to Philadelphia, Gerhard put his new skills to ready use during a typhoid outbreak in 1837, when he published an article that constituted a large step in differentiating between typhoid and typhus fevers, diseases that resembled one another, especially in the extent and nature of their rashes.[10] Gerhard was cofounder of a scientific journal, *Medical Examiner*, which he edited for years, and he accepted a professorship at the University of Pennsylvania. Through his lectures and writing, Gerhard educated a generation of America's top medical talent in Philadelphia and beyond.

Compared to the hospitals and pathology rooms of Paris, to say nothing of the rounds of lectures American students attended throughout the day and far into the evening in Paris, even America's medical center, Philadelphia, seemed almost anti-intellectual. At least a portion of the newfound disdain with which some Parisian-educated Philadelphia physicians viewed the city's medical establishment resulted from haughty self-importance acquired from their experience in Paris. Upon his return to Philadelphia, Alfred Stille wrote to a fellow physician that "the true spirit of scientific research . . . can hardly be said to exist here."[11] In their shared disdain for the seeming backwardness of medicine in even Philadelphia, Paris-educated physicians drew close and even closed ranks on their fellow doctors. In the case of Philadelphia, this culminated in seizing the reins of the College of Physicians from men who did not experience, and had not accepted, the new methods that men like Gerhard and Stille imported from Europe.[12] Yet in the midst of its triumph over older forms of orthodox medicine, the new, Parisian-based model of medicine provoked a backlash from physicians and laypeople who objected to the reduction of patients to mere research material and who perceived in the Paris model, and those Americans it schooled, a lack of emphasis on healing in preference for esoteric understanding of disease processes.[13]

As old forms of disease causation and treatment lost their hold, and few new treatments from regular physicians emerged, a variety of alternative theories of health and medicine emerged. Homeopathy was the best known and most powerful of the non-allopathic, or unconventional, schools of medicine. Devised by a German doctor, Samuel Hahnemann, homeopathy operated under the theory that minute doses of substances that caused symptoms like those produced by particular diseases and disorders allowed the body to overcome illness. To put it succinctly, homeopathy is based on a wholly unscientific notion that "like defeats like." Homeopathy fashioned a powerful base of practitioners, schools, and hospitals in eastern Pennsylvania, and its popularity made it a national phenomenon. The first medical school in the world dedicated to homeopathy was founded in 1835 in Allentown by three leading lights in homeopathic medical circles, including Constantine Hering, a man widely considered a father of homeopathy in America.[14] The North American Academy of the Homeopathic Healing Art, as the school was named, lasted a mere six years and then closed in 1841, its teaching mission taken up in 1848 by the far more famous Homeopathic Medical College of Pennsylvania, located in Philadelphia and also opened by Hering.[15] The Homeopathic Medical College opened a teaching hospital just a few years later, later renamed Hahnemann Hospital.

Another important therapeutic school, hydrotherapy or water cure, was introduced to Pennsylvania in the 1830s from Europe. People who selected the water-cure method drank a variety of plain and mineral waters, indulged in hot and cold baths, and used enemas and other water-based treatments. Water-cure "doctors" avoided the use of most caustic chemicals, mercury, and opium but also generally disdained more innocuous substances like coffee and tea.[16] Practitioners opened water-cure hospitals throughout the state, and by midcentury the clinics proved so popular that almost every county in Pennsylvania possessed at least one water-cure hospital, most of which were located along watercourses or springs that bubbled from the state's limestone. One of the state's more famous hydropathic hospitals opened in 1846 in Fountain Hill, Lehigh County, about sixty miles outside Philadelphia.[17] The basis for the hospital, named the Bethlehem Hydropathic Institute, was a spring that percolated near the top of the South Mountain Ridge. The institute treated patients for a quarter century until insolvency closed it. By the 1860s, dozens of water-cure hotels and resorts dotted the state, many of them situated on springs, though within a decade many had closed as people increasingly turned to allopathic and homeopathic medicine for treatment.

Even as new forms of medical practice staked their claim in Pennsylvania's medical marketplace, practices that dated to the colonial era remained robust. Most medicine during the early republic and antebellum periods took place in the home. This rule applied even when serious disease or major trauma was present. Powwowing is an example of a practice that remained popular. From the large concentrations of powwowers in the eastern third of the state where powwowing first took root in the eighteenth century, it spread to communities in central Pennsylvania and may have hit its zenith during the first half of the nineteenth century. Though it will never be possible to ascertain the number of powwow doctors in Pennsylvania, it is likely that thousands claimed the power, through powwowing, to heal the sick. Most powwowers practiced informally, with family and friends their only patients. Others practiced openly in the community as powwowers, their services sought by friend and stranger alike. In 1820, the most famous powwow text, *The Long Lost Friend*, was published by a Reading powwow doctor, John George Hohman.[18] Reprinted for decades—including updated editions—*The Long Lost Friend* offered prayers, remedies, and advice to those who wished to heal through powwow. Hohman's work also marked the single greatest act of commercialization of the practice since its development more than a century earlier.

In addition to the numerous homeopathic and water-cure clinics that blossomed in the state, a number of conventional hospitals opened in the decades before the Civil War. All of the new hospitals were founded in Philadelphia and Pittsburgh, a product of the wealth concentration and population density of those cities. A socioreligious motivation also underlay the wave of hospital construction during the first half of the nineteenth century; elites publicly showed their Christian charity to the less fortunate through founding hospitals.[19] Despite the charitable intentions of founders and managers, nineteenth-century sensibilities informed who could be admitted and under what circumstances. Both public and private institutions wished to avoid becoming tenements for the poor and often required that a respectable member of local society vouch for a prospective patient's moral soundness. Hospital managers routinely excluded alcoholics, unwed mothers, and assorted other notorious characters, a practice in keeping with the period's division of the destitute into the "deserving" and "undeserving" poor.

The Thomas Jefferson University Hospital opened in 1825, and while its wards and surgical rooms offered competent care to the sick and injured, it also enhanced the medical education of students at Jefferson Medical College. In 1855, an important specialist hospital, Children's Hospital of Philadelphia, opened with twelve beds and an outpatient dispensary for the city's sick and injured youngsters. Children's Hospital offered treatment free of charge and aimed to fill an important gap in the city's health care; the children of the poor often suffered and died for simple want of medical treatment. Another specialty hospital, the Friends Hospital, opened in 1813 to serve another underserved group, those with psychological and emotional problems. The Friends Hospital operated under a philosophy that offered dignity to its patients, not the prison-like conditions in which most institutionalized people lived.

In Pittsburgh, the influx of Catholic immigrants prompted religious orders to open hospitals. Private hospitals were especially important to Pittsburgh because the city founded few public hospitals, apart from a pest house and tuberculosis farm, to treat a population that faced terrible injuries and rampant disease in the city's growing industrial works and the poor neighborhoods that surrounded them. In 1847, the Sisters of Mercy founded the city's first hospital, Mercy Hospital, for the poor, especially Irish laborers with little money for physicians.[20] Two years later, the Pittsburgh Infirmary, later expanded and renamed Passavant Hospital, opened its doors under the auspices of the Lutheran Church and became the first Protestant hospital in the country.[21] The first nondenominational hospital charted in Pittsburgh was Western Pennsylvania Hospital, which opened in 1853 and grew steadily through the end of the nineteenth century.[22]

The expansion of Pennsylvania's medical capabilities notwithstanding, medicine remained a conservative discipline. The experience of Elizabeth Blackwell, the first woman to earn a medical degree in the United States, is instructive. Born in 1821, Blackwell earned her medical degree at Geneva College in New York, in 1849. After her first year of medical studies, Blackwell took a position at Blockley Almshouse in Philadelphia to hone her skills as a clinician. Blackwell was shocked by conditions in the institution. Paupers who resided at Blockley worked as nurses and aides in the hospital. Untrained and with little reason to care about their charges, the resident attendants often abused or ignored patients, which added to the chaotic, overcrowded conditions in Blockley. Blackwell's status as a female physician in training did not endear her to most of her male colleagues. While many of the women nurses treated her as a professional, Blackwell wrote that "the young resident physicians . . . were not friendly. When I walked into the wards they walked out."[23] To make her rounds even more difficult—to say nothing of compromising patient care—Blackwell observed that the male physicians "ceased to write the diagnosis and treatment of patients on the card at the head of each bed . . . thus throwing me entirely on my own resources for clinical study."[24]

Though the hidebound nature of gender relations in Pennsylvania medicine inflicted numerous indignities on Blackwell, her time at Blockley proved an invaluable addition to her medical education. Blackwell treated patients on the wards dedicated to women infected with syphilis. Syphilis, the most deadly sexually transmitted disease of the nineteenth century, slowly ate away at soft tissue and possessed the propensity for causing severe neurological symptoms, including mood changes, sudden violent outbursts, and insanity. Blackwell admitted that until her time on the syphilis wards, she was "strangely ignorant . . . of the selfish relations of men and women."[25] It came as a deep shock that "most of the women are unmarried, a large proportion having lived at service and been seduced by their masters," and were then left to rot, literally, in a poorhouse.[26] Blackwell's feminism was influenced by her time among Philadelphia's poorest syphilitic women. An experience even more pertinent to her medical education was her thesis, "Ship Fever: An Inaugural Thesis," the foundation of which was her work with Irish immigrants at Blockley. Blackwell believed that the ship fever from which the recent immigrants suffered was a "form of typhus," and that she was fortunate to be "studying in the midst of the poor dying sufferers who crowded the hospital wards."[27]

Toward a Scientific Standard

One of the great themes of medicine in Pennsylvania throughout the nineteenth century was the movement to professionalize medical education and practice along conventional scientific lines, which included the use of drugs—pharmaceuticals—to treat disease. For the conventional doctor, practitioners of the water cure, homeopathy, and the like were no better than the manufacturers of patent medicine whose concoctions made their inventors fortunes, but whose curative properties were nil. For their part, homeopaths and water-cure healers, in addition to the great number of powwow and other sorts of faith healers, were adamant that their methods not only were effective but presented less risk to patients than many of the standard treatments advanced by allopathic medicine.

The confidence patients placed in non-allopathic treatments reveals a complex relation between patient preferences and the efficacy, or lack of efficacy, of both irregular and conventional medical practices. Importantly, with the exception of smallpox vaccination, conventional medicine during the antebellum period offered little reliable empirical evidence for its power to prevent or cure infectious disease. While the same was true for powwowing, homeopathy, and water cures, such unconventional treatments did not inflict additional discomfort on their users. Furthermore, beyond the power of suggestion—the placebo effect—unconventional medicine did offer patients comfort, as well as some confirmation of the effectiveness of their treatment regimes. For instance, immersion in warm and cold baths cleaned and refreshed patients, and hot water and mineral salts eased aches and pains—and convinced the patient of the potency of water-cure therapy during a period when, beyond opium, conventional medicine offered little to assuage pain.

Furthermore, homeopathy and other schools of irregular medicine did important work "in protesting the too-heroic character" of regular medicine.[28]

Unfortunately for irregular practitioners, their theories and therapies remained static even as regular practitioners continuously benefited from the power of science to forge new understandings of disease, prevention, and cure. While the pace of scientific advances, and their practical effect, remained small throughout the antebellum period, the foundations of conventional medicine's future dominance of the state's public health and medical markets were laid by 1860. One of the pillars of that foundation was the half dozen medical schools founded in Philadelphia before the Civil War. While all of Pennsylvania's medical schools before 1866 were located in Philadelphia, the doctors they trained moved beyond the city and slowly improved medicine throughout the state. Over the course of the nineteenth century, medical schools' curricula became more technical as the expertise required to earn a degree in medicine grew increasingly esoteric and lengthy. Jefferson Medical College, which opened in 1824, was the most prestigious of the schools that joined the University of Pennsylvania's medical school. The founding of Jefferson was even more important to the education of the state's medical elite as the University of Pennsylvania's medical program went into a decades-long decline that lasted from the 1830s through midcentury.[29]

A more notable new medical school, the Women's Medical College of Pennsylvania, founded in 1850, was the second medical school for women in the country. In 1861, the Women's Medical Hospital opened its doors and, like its counterpart hospitals at Penn and Jefferson, offered students at the Women's Medical College the same sort of clinical experience from which men routinely profited. Reflecting on the importance of clinical training to the advancement of women in the medical profession more than thirty years later, Frances Emily White, a professor at the Women's Medical College, suggested that "the chief disadvantages from which medical women in this country now suffer arise from their exclusion from the work of the great public hospitals" during their training.[30]

The first African American woman to attend medical school in the United States, Sarah Mapps Douglass, attended the school in the early 1850s, though she did not graduate.[31] In 1867, the Women's Medical College graduated the second African American physician in the nation, Rebecca J. Cole, who practiced medicine in South Carolina and Philadelphia.[32] That the college offered African American women a way forward in medicine was important, but equally important was the general effect of the college, which remained for decades one of a small handful of schools to offer medical degrees to women regardless of color or station in life. Furthermore, though the nine-teenth century saw scores of medical colleges open their doors and grant degrees to men after a scant course of studies, the Women's Medical College, perhaps because of its location in one of the nation's medical capitals, was noted for its excellent education and strong laboratory facilities. By the end of the century it offered a course of study on a par, in many ways, with Johns Hopkins University.[33]

Of even more immediate importance to the trend of medical profession-alization and standardization in Pennsylvania than medical schools were the dozen county medical societies founded before the Civil War. The societies varied in quality, and about half were concentrated within one hundred miles of Philadelphia, but all of the societies aimed to educate local physicians and empower them politically, and usually accepted for membership only those physicians who practiced regular medicine. In 1847, the American Medical Association was founded in Philadelphia, partly in response to the prolifera-tion of unorthodox medical practices.[34] A year later the state's doctors founded an organization that grew far more powerful than any of the county societies—the Medical Society of Pennsylvania. The state medical society worked to knit together not individual doctors but the county medical soci-eties, and absolutely no irregular physicians were allowed to join the society.[35] Furthermore, during the 1850s, the society ruled that members should not associate with irregular doctors.

It was for this reason that the society repeatedly, albeit disingenuously, affirmed the right of women to practice medicine, and that the society would happily accept women for membership, were it not for the fact that women's medical schools employed large numbers of irregular practitioners as profes-sors.[36] Women, then, suffered a de facto ban on their membership in the state medical society and concentrated their healing efforts among the state's new-borns, children, and women. The society delivered a final major blow against irregular medicine when it demanded that society members absolutely ab-stain from entering into business associations with apothecaries, as such re-lationships not only violated the code of ethics promulgated by the society but also endangered the public because, the society suggested, many apothe-caries proffered only nostrums.[37]

Within a generation of its founding, the society emerged as a fierce, and politically connected, lobby in Harrisburg that by the late nineteenth century pressured the state legislature and a series of governors to enact medical and public health reforms. Almost without exception the most prestigious physi-cians in Pennsylvania joined the society and, though Philadelphia's physi-cians, many of them with a strong research background, tended to dominate

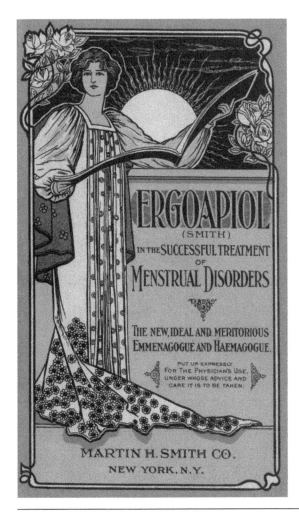

Advertisement for Ergoapiol, 1904. Patent medicine came increasingly under fire from conventional medical societies. Medicines such as this one, produced by Martin H. Smith Company, aimed to reduce menstrual symptoms and various other "ailments" that afflicted women but often contained dangerous ingredients, such as morphine mixed with alcohol. (Courtesy of the College of Physicians of Philadelphia.)

the society's direction, the executive committee perennially included medical leaders from even the state's most rural districts. For sixty years, the society tried to enforce some sort of standard on the state's medical profession when the state refused to set even the mildest guidelines. The society's annual meetings offered doctors far removed from major hospitals and universities the opportunity to further their medical education as new research and medical instruments were explained during the lecture series component of the meetings. The Medical Society of Pennsylvania also forged links beyond the commonwealth, as its leadership met with members of other states' medical societies, especially the county and state medical societies of New Jersey. Pennsylvania furthered cemented its connections with physicians and sanitarians across the nation when, in 1857, the Philadelphia board of health hosted a national sanitary convention in Philadelphia.[38]

The Civil War

Epidemics, noted one historian, are events, not trends, and thus expose fault lines in medicine and public health.[39] Wars, too, are events that highlight the capabilities and limitations in medicine at a particular moment in history. The American Civil War occurred at a curious time in the history of American medicine, when improvements in a variety of medical fields combined with a still-muddled understanding of how infectious diseases spread and, of course, the role of pathogens in causing disease in the first place. As a result, the wounded and sick experienced a better sort of military medicine than their predecessors had during the American Revolution, the War of 1812, and even the Mexican-American War, scarcely a dozen years past. Yet sepsis was common and untreatable, gangrene uniformly resulted in either amputation or death, and the camp diseases that killed at Valley Forge in 1778 carried off tens of thousands of soldiers during the Civil War.

Surgery had always been hampered by two factors; infection often set in and killed the patient even if the surgery was successful, and surgery inflicted excruciating pain on the patient. A Civil War surgeon could do little about infection, but two new substances did allow a doctor to render surgeries painless. In Scotland, doctors began to use chloroform during the mid-1840s as a general anesthetic. Almost simultaneously, doctors in Boston introduced ether as an anesthetic for surgery. By the Civil War, both substances were readily available to military doctors, though the Union produced its own supplies of the drugs, much of it manufactured in Philadelphia, while the South needed to import them through the blockade. General anesthesia revolutionized the surgical experience for both patient and doctor. The patient did not thrash about in agony, which made the surgeon's job less difficult; fewer surgical patients died of shock; and surgeons were not forced to rush to spare their patients pain. Still, postoperative pain control was largely the domain of opium solutions and willpower on the part of patients. Also, use of ether and chloroform could lead to death because administering a lethal dose was relatively easy, though surgeons recorded few cases of overdose during the war.

Despite losses on the battlefield and by wounds inflicted during battle, most of America's losses during the war occurred as a result of disease, a state of affairs that did not change until World War II. Camps, especially large camps that housed tens of thousands of soldiers, were incredibly unsanitary.

Excrement from men and horses fouled nearby water sources just as they did in cities, which resulted in widespread gastrointestinal illness, mostly typhoid and dysentery. Measles, too, took a heavy toll, as did diphtheria, influenza, and pneumonia. Fortunately, the war did not coincide with another cholera pandemic and the armies managed to avoid that scourge. Complicating the gastrointestinal dangers of camp life were the abysmal rations served to the men, typically salted meat and biscuits, often spoiled and poorly cooked. Soldiers consumed almost no fresh fruit or vegetables, which contributed to scurvy and other nutritive deficiencies. Even worse, most of the fighting occurred in the South, where the warm climate and plentiful standing water encouraged breeding populations of mosquitoes that carried malaria.

In that face of what appeared to be insurmountable obstacles to health, defenses were fashioned that mitigated some of the threats, and Pennsylvania played a key role. Dr. Samuel D. Gross, born near Easton, Pennsylvania, and educated at Jefferson Medical College, spent decades before the Civil War refining medical techniques and education along the lines of the Paris model.[40] In only nine days at the very beginning of the war, he wrote a "pocket manual" of surgery specifically for the Union Army. The guide circulated widely and was eventually used by surgeons in the Confederate Army too. Of even greater importance was the work of Dr. Jonathan Letterman. Born in Canonsburg, in the southwestern portion of the state, Letterman graduated from Jefferson Medical College in 1848 and immediately entered the army as a surgeon.[41] His service before the Civil War was spent on the frontier, seemingly always engaged in one of the endless wars against various Native American groups and in the rough forts that dotted the western territories. In 1862, General George B. McClellan appointed him medical director of the Army of the Potomac, the major formation engaged in fighting General Robert E. Lee in the area around Washington, D.C., and Richmond, Virginia.

The first task Letterman undertook was the organization of an ambulance corps. The ambulance corps was responsible for not only removing men to hospitals but also removing wounded men from the battlefield itself. Next, Letterman turned to the amount and variety of supplies carried into the field by the surgeons and physicians of the Army of the Potomac. He found that "the quantity of these materials carried was often excessive, and in other cases insufficient."[42] He therefore reduced the quantities of most of the medicines and equipment and thereby reduced the number of horse teams and wagons required to haul medical supplies. Finally, Letterman issued a set of orders covering the function and form of field hospitals in the Army of the Potomac, a novel idea adopted by the entire Union Army. Letterman's "scheme of organization" was designed as an interlocking system that facilitated quick removal of the wounded from the battlefield by the ambulance corps to field hospitals whose organization and purpose were standardized, and whose treatment of the wounded was made better by a ready and rational stock of supplies.[43]

Pennsylvania's civilians played an important role in caring for the wounded and ameliorating the awful conditions found in the army's cantonments. The largest and best known of the efforts were the sanitary fairs, which were an outgrowth of the United States Sanitary Commission. The USSC was an umbrella organization that brought together volunteers, citizens groups, churches, and money for the purpose of caring for Union troops while they were in camp or hospital. Sanitary fairs were designed to enlist the support of civilians by harnessing their patriotism toward a practical end. Fairgoers purchased tickets and bought items at the fair, the money designated for the purchase of items for the benefit of soldiers in the field—for instance, bedding and bandages. Donated money also underwrote inspection trips by USSC representatives to army camps and hospitals in an attempt to improve sanitary conditions and paid for the removal of the wounded to hospitals in Philadelphia and other cities.

The greatest of the fairs, the Great Central Fair, was held for three weeks in Logan Square in Philadelphia during June 1864, when visitors purchased almost a half million tickets. In the weeks leading up to the fair, a fundraising committee toured the populous sections of eastern Pennsylvania and urged people to donate a day's wages to the construction of the fairgrounds; in short order more than a quarter million dollars was raised. The fairgrounds stretched over many acres and included a massive arch more than five hundred feet long and specially designed buildings whose ceilings admitted the branches of the trees that grew in Logan Square and created "an unusual effect."[44] The fanfare of the great Philadelphia sanitary fair provoked an outpouring of financial support that totaled more than a million dollars. Perhaps the most striking aspect of the fairs in Philadelphia and Pittsburgh, as well as those in other major cities, was their purpose; the fairs made up for the very basic, and glaring, deficiencies in the medical and sanitary services of the military and were not simply a form of nineteenth-century care packages that many individuals and organizations send to American military personnel in the twenty-first century. Put in this light, the Great Sanitary Fair and smaller fairs contributed mightily to the health of the Union Army.

The worst mass casualty incident in Pennsylvania during the mid-nineteenth century was the Battle of Gettysburg, the deadliest confrontation in a war noted for its violence. By one account more than thirty thousand wounded lay waiting for care in the homes, churches, and businesses of Gettysburg, while others were warehoused in tents on the edge of the battlefield, surrounded by men hideously wounded and dying.[45] To transport and tend the men, Letterman's medical corps assembled a thousand ambulances, 650 medical officers, and more than three thousand stretcher bearers and drivers.[46] Every sort of medical discipline treated the injured in the days and weeks after the battle; though allopathic medicine was the official medicine of the Union forces, large numbers of civilian doctors both entered the army and converged on the battlefield from their civilian practices and employed their preferred modes of treatment.[47]

On their approach to the town the volunteers all noticed a stench so overwhelming that one nurse from New Jersey remembered it as a "sickening, overpowerful, awful stench."[48] A little girl from the town remembered the odor was worse than "the time we found a dead rat behind the loose boards in the cellar."[49] Even soldiers inured to the aftermath of major battles vomited uncontrollably and remained unable to eat for days. Among the rotting bodies lay men so injured they could not crawl to safety. Once the wounded reached the temporary hospitals, violent thunderstorms on July 4 raised streams above their banks and filled low places on the battlefield, including some of the hospitals, and drowned many of the wounded. Clouds of flies produced by the corpses harried everyone while hogs roamed the killing fields eating the dead and attacking the injured, with one civilian in Gettysburg remarking years later that "numerous rough boxes" for the dead lay near a road.[50] The volunteers did not relent and tried to organize the wounded for transport to larger hospitals in nearby cities.

Many of the civilian doctors and nurses were horrified by not just the wounds they saw, but the number of amputations surgeons performed. Months later, hundreds of soldiers lay convalescing in the state's hospitals, especially in Philadelphia, while temporary military hospitals were erected alongside already existing civilian hospitals. No other northern state's medical resources were involved as directly in the war effort as those of Pennsylvania, in large part because the commonwealth lay adjacent to the battlefields of northern Virginia but also because, whether at war or peace, the state was the center of medicine in the United States.[51]

Conclusion

Pennsylvania medicine spent much of the early nineteenth century little better equipped to fight disease and improve the lot of its citizens than the colonial medicine of the eighteenth century. A closer examination, however, reveals that Pennsylvania medicine embarked on a series of transitions in its intellectual approach to disease and health, as well as making strides in the commonwealth's medical infrastructure. Importantly, the absolute success, as measured by scientific correctness, of portions of the transition is not the best way to judge the era. For instance, unorthodox schools of medical thought, most importantly water cure and homeopathy, may at first appear as missteps in the overall scientific progress of humanity against disease. However, both disciplines were part of a growing rejection of older forms of medicine increasingly seen as ineffective by all medical doctrines, both allopathic and unorthodox.

Turning away from the most extreme forms of bleeding and purging occurred across the entirety of medical thought, and thus momentum built and space was carved for consideration of other forms of medicine. The most crucial development in the intellectual milieu of medicine in the first half of the nineteenth century was the growing effort to standardize and refine, on a scientific basis, conventional medicine. Medical schools certainly contributed to the push, but even more important in the early phases were the founding of the state and county medical societies. The societies enforced an intellectual discipline on their members and increasingly demanded that members make a choice between either eschewing unorthodox medicine and joining county societies, or abandoning the access to resources and respect that membership in medical societies entailed. Changes in medical thought did not happen overnight, and many members of medical societies practiced medicine that included elements of the allopathic and the unconventional, but a march toward scientific uniformity was well under way by 1860.

The early nineteenth century was also important for the new foundation of medicine-as-science. While few cures emerged, discarding old ideas of pathology and cures prepared "the only basis upon which a succeeding generation could at last build a systematic structure of prevention and cure."[52] The tedious construction of a new medical science that increasingly admitted the errors of past suppositions about disease and cures contrasted sharply with the irregular schools of medicine that believed "all diseases were really simply this and that" and that a single cure, which always depended on the ideas of the sect in question, sufficed.[53] In short, supporters of the allopathic school of medicine spent much of the early nineteenth century rejecting their own precepts and forging a new understanding of disease and treatment while practitioners of the irregular schools evinced little or no impulse toward the sort of experimentation required to further their understanding of disease and cures. As long as allopaths could offer few or no effective treatments, irregular schools of medical thought often prevailed in their struggle for patients, fees, and respect. However, when scientific medicine moved on from its own overarching theories of disease causation, for instance miasma, and cure-all treatments like bleeding and purging in favor of causation and treatments based on observation in both clinical and laboratory settings, irregular medical sects that failed to follow suit could not help but undermine their own credibility.

The medical infrastructure of the state had also increased dramatically by the time of the Civil War. As in the intellectual battles fought between the various medical factions, Pennsylvania's health infrastructure did not follow a single, clear line. Instead, hospitals and clinics that represented every sort of medical theory emerged throughout the state. Water-cure clinics and hospitals were easily the most numerous, in large measure because water clinics required nothing more complicated or expensive than a building and access to copious amounts of water. Homeopathic hospitals and conventional hospitals were more sophisticated and expensive, and it comes as no surprise both were concentrated in the state's cities and large towns, with conventional hospitals wholly confined to Philadelphia and Pittsburgh. Likewise, the medical school established by homeopathic practitioners and the additional two allopathic schools founded during the period found their homes in the wealthy and educated cities. By the end of the Civil War, Pennsylvania emerged as America's most important industrialized state, while the state's medicine was perched on the cusp of an era of massive expansion.

3

TRIUMPH OF THE ALLOPATHS, 1866–1905

THE LAST FOUR DECADES of the nineteenth century were the most important in medical history. Indeed, the basis for modern medicine stretches to discoveries that emerged during the era. The current of scientific innovation not only swept Pennsylvania along but was strengthened by the state's scientists, hospitals, and laboratories. Much of the important medical research done in the state emerged from Philadelphia's universities and hospitals. But hospitals in even very obscure locations in Pennsylvania did much practical good by founding nursing schools that helped revolutionize hospital care among the state's rural population, a demographic that constituted the majority of the state's residents and had few alternatives for treatment beyond local healers and country doctors. Pennsylvania also began the process of building the capacity to protect the public's health by founding a state board of health. By 1905, the frustrating history of the state board of health closed when the legislature and governor inaugurated a state department of health that quickly grew into the strongest, most competent health department in the country.

The Bacterial Revolution

The last forty years of the nineteenth century witnessed a fundamental change in the biological sciences—the bacterial revolution. Bacteriology was an entirely new path of investigation that ascribed to microbes causation for infectious disease. The new knowledge led to the development of increasingly effective medical and public health tools to control and even cure disease. Louis Pasteur is often credited with initiating the age of bacteriology in the late 1850s and 1860s by studying the action of yeast and bacteria in the wine-making process. His observations led Pasteur to the conclusion that when heated, most bacteria and yeast are rendered inactive or dead. He applied what he learned to the food supply and showed that beer, and most importantly milk, could be heated, killing bacteria and thereby slowing spoilage and reducing human illness. The process is termed pasteurization. By the early 1860s, Pasteur disproved the notion that life could spontaneously spring from decaying matter. His research suggested that anything that grew in rotting tissue was the result of being carried onto and into it by insects, the air, and other means. Finally, Pasteur also largely proved that bacteria might be weakened by exposure to oxygen or heat yet still provoke immunity in animals into which they were injected.

In Scotland, a physician at the Glasgow Infirmary, Joseph Lister, avidly followed Pasteur's work in the scientific journals. Lister began to connect Pasteur's refutation of the theory of spontaneous generation with his own suspicions about wound infection. In short, Lister believed that wound infection was akin to fermentation, a process that required yeast and bacteria. Furthermore, he discovered that railroad ties dipped in a coal tar derivative called carbolic acid resisted rot for years, though no one knew why. Lister experimented by dousing surgical instruments, his hands, and other equipment in the acid, a regime which seemed to lower infections among his patients. In 1865, Lister treated a boy who sustained a compound fracture of his lower leg. In such cases, a stark choice presented itself; a physician could either amputate or set the bone, close the wound, and wait for the almost inevitable infection to set in and then either amputate or watch as the patient died of septicemia. Lister rejected both alternatives and instead set the bone, placed a carbolic acid–soaked cloth in the wound, and kept the wound open. After six weeks of replacing the cloth every few days, the bone healed, and the wound closed without complications from infection. When Lister published his results in 1867, the antiseptic revolution in surgery and wound care was initiated.

In Germany, a physician with a genius for research and experimentation, Robert Koch, suspected that the microbes he and others detected under the microscope were responsible for causing contagious disease. In 1878, Koch proved that anthrax in sheep was caused by a bacterium he isolated from the blood of diseased sheep. In March 1882 Koch stunned the world when he announced that a method for staining bacteria allowed him to isolate the bacterium responsible for causing tuberculosis. In one fell swoop Koch not only identified a pathogen responsible for causing disease in humans but also succeeded in unmasking the cause of the deadliest disease in Europe and North America. In just the twenty years following Koch's confirmation of bacteria's role in tuberculosis, scientists identified the pathogens responsible for causing diphtheria, tetanus, cholera, typhoid, plague, scarlet fever, and pneumococcal pneumonia.

Confirmation of bacteria's causative role in infectious disease did not force an incremental change in the way humanity understood disease. Instead, a common understanding that germs were the cause of disease meant that science had finally pierced, once and for all, the mystery of infectious disease. Medicine now held the requisite knowledge for working toward effective treatments. Public health efforts based on the new science of bacteriology now stood a reasonable chance of shielding people from disease through updated versions of isolation and quarantine, water filtration, and other methods. As the science of medicine, both in the laboratory and the clinic, produced a seemingly endless stream of new knowledge concerning microbes, it seemed certain that new vaccines would emerge, like those available for smallpox in humans and anthrax in sheep, to protect people from illness. Little more than a decade later, in late 1892, an antitoxin for use against diphtheria debuted, its power to rally the body's immune system against diphtheria so great that it may fairly be termed the first "silver bullet" against infection. At roughly the same time, an antitoxin was developed for use against tetanus, and medicine promised even greater benefits in the future.

In Pennsylvania, medical schools most fully felt the effects of European innovations. Throughout the mid- to late nineteenth century, training in even the best American medical schools lagged behind their European counterparts. American medical students continued, as they had for decades, to travel to universities and hospitals in Great Britain, France, Germany, and Austria to study the newest theories and practices. Returning students and physicians brought with them new ideas about the standard of training physicians should receive, the function of hospitals, the role of nurses, and how public health is best managed. The University of Pennsylvania's medical school absorbed the new methods of instruction before other medical programs did, and by the mid-1880s, it counted among its faculty a number of leaders in their respective fields, including Joseph Leidy in anatomy, William Osler in clinical medicine, and William Pepper in theory and practice.[1]

Under the leadership of these men, and in conformity with the practices of European universities, Penn opened its biology department under the supervision of Leidy in 1885 and in 1889 opened the first hygiene laboratory in the nation under the direction of Samuel G. Dixon, a newly appointed pro-

fessor in the school of medicine.[2] Jefferson Medical College, too, strengthened its program of study by retaining physicians like Wilmer Krusen as
professor of gynecology and John C. Da Costa, a professor of medicine and
the editor of an American edition of *Gray's Anatomy*.

The number of medical schools in Pennsylvania expanded by only two
during the Gilded Age and Progressive Era; Western Pennsylvania Medical
College opened its doors in 1887 and became the medical school of the University of Pittsburgh in 1908. While the founders of Western Pennsylvania
Medical College intended to give Pittsburgh a solid medical school of its own,
it remained a minor school in terms of standards and faculty until almost
World War I, a process explored in Chapter 4. Very late in the period, 1901,
Temple University inaugurated its medical school. Temple's program broke
new ground as the first coeducational medical program in America. Classes
met at night to accommodate its targeted student population of striving, but
not affluent, working people, which included Jews, Catholics, and African
Americans. Temple's liberal admittance policies and evening classes drew the
ire of the city's physicians, who feared that the medical degree in the hands
of Temple would be less valuable. Temple assuaged some of these concerns
when, a few years later, the university ended night classes. Medical education,
therefore, remained concentrated in Philadelphia, highly conventional from
a sociocultural perspective, and increasingly scientifically esoteric.

Two institutions dedicated to the education of African American physicians were also founded during the period. The first was at Lincoln University
in Oxford, Chester County. Founded in 1854 as the country's first histori-
cally black college, Lincoln founded its medical school in 1870.[3] After just
four years in operation, the medical school closed and its students either
pursued other career paths or found a home in medical programs that accepted people of color. Twenty years after Lincoln closed its doors to medical
students, the Frederick Douglass Memorial Hospital and Training School
opened. The hospital was the first to serve the African American community,
though it accepted patients regardless "of creed or color, or because they are
too poor to pay."[4] The founder, Nathan Francis Mossell, was the first African
American to earn his medical degree from the University of Pennsylvania, in
1882, and broke new ground in 1888 when his colleagues elected him a
member of the Philadelphia Medical Society.

After Mossell opened a private practice on Lombard Street, "at the center
of the city's black belt," he saw the need for a hospital to treat African American patients and later wrote that though the hospital "has been embarrassed
financially; [it] has continued faith however in the final triumph of righteous-
ness."[5] In addition to treating patients, the hospital functioned as a place

where African American doctors could gain clinical experience, especially during the early phases of their medical education. The hospital also trained black nurses, who otherwise saw their opportunities limited. Overall, Douglass Memorial earned the respect of Philadelphia's most progressive and influential physicians, many of whom endeavored to aid it politically and financially.

Until well into the twentieth century, breakthroughs in medicine generally flowed from east to west across the Atlantic. A notable insight credited to a Pennsylvania scientist involved the founder of the University of Pennsylvania's hygiene laboratory, Samuel Dixon. Throughout his career Dixon concentrated on tuberculosis and, in 1889, was the first to prove that tuberculosis could be attenuated (weakened) by exposure to temperature changes.[6] Capitalizing on his discovery, Dixon published evidence that old cultures of tuberculosis bacteria, when introduced into test animals, provoked some degree of immunity. By 1890, Dixon devised an extract from attenuated tuberculosis bacteria that hindered the growth of tubercular lesions in animals and humans.[7] A minor controversy occurred when Koch, discoverer of the organism responsible for tuberculosis, claimed he attenuated tuberculosis before Dixon. A transatlantic meeting of scientific minds resolved the matter in Dixon's favor. In the case of immune-producing extracts, which Dixon and Koch created independently of one another's research, Koch's proved a colossal failure that killed many patients before its use was discontinued, while Dixon's serum was used by physicians even decades later to ameliorate glandular, genitourinary, and ocular tuberculosis. Along similar lines, Albert C. Barnes, another graduate of Penn's medical school, developed a silver nitrate antiseptic used to treat both genital gonorrhea in adults and ocular gonorrhea in newborns.

Scientific discoveries not only increased the potency of allopathic medicine; they also undermined the credibility of non-allopathic schools of medicine. At least part of the power of unconventional practitioners, be they herbalists, powwowers, water-cure doctors, or homeopaths, was derived from the inability of regular practitioners to offer adequate treatments. As science unlocked the role of bacteria in disease and worked out progressively better techniques to prevent and cure disease, irregular healers proved unable to offer either reasonable explanations for disease causation or treatments that grew more effective. Increasingly, alternative healers became just that: an alternative to conventional medicine. By 1900, conventional medicine managed to push most unorthodox healers and their theories ever further from the realm of the plausible and into the domain of the quack doctor and patent elixir. As a result, the water-cure clinic virtually disappeared by the 1890s.

Homeopaths, too, saw their domain shrink on a national level by the end of the nineteenth century, but Pennsylvania, and especially the Lehigh Valley and Philadelphia, remained homeopathy's primary "bastion of strength" in the United States.[8] The ostracism of homeopaths from medical societies, medical schools, and hospitals continued, but the state's medical licensing laws did not place onerous burdens on homeopathic practitioners.

The fate of powwowing in the late nineteenth century was a more straightforward affair connected not only to advances in medicine but, perhaps even more importantly, to a world transformed by industrialization. New factories and mills sprouted in the formerly agricultural villages and towns of the heavily Pennsylvania Dutch counties of Berks, Lancaster, Lebanon, Lehigh, Schuylkill, and York, drawing hundreds of thousands of workers and their families, many of them not Pennsylvania German. Larger towns like Bethlehem, Allentown, and Reading added tens of thousands to their populations between 1870 and 1900 and grew into small cities. The region's new wealth built colleges and universities, founded hospitals, and fostered a new intellectualism based on science.

Powwowing seemed an archaic relic of the past that served only to harm the region's image.[9] Newspapers, especially in Allentown and Reading, but also nationally, chronicled the exploits of local powwowers, whom the newspapers often referred to as "witch doctors" or "witches," while people who enlisted powwowers were characterized as "ignorant" souls who needed to "break off the shackles of the 'dark ages.'"[10] The travails of one powwower, "Doctor" Henry Grate, were chronicled by Allentown's newspapers for decades. Grate earned frequent jail terms and even beatings at the hands of irate husbands whose wives parted with large sums of money for nostrums and spells.[11] By 1900 powwowing almost entirely disappeared from the region's cities if only because local authorities fined and jailed practitioners for fraud and practicing medicine without a license, while urban residents increasingly eschewed powwowers' services. Dwindling numbers of powwow healers practiced in small rural communities whose people both respected powwow's ability to heal and often feared its perceived ability to bewitch. Yet even as many forms of non-allopathic medicine ebbed in the late nineteenth century, new folk medicine brought to Pennsylvania by new immigrants began to flourish and even combined with powwowing.[12]

The eastern anthracite region exemplifies the blending of myriad strains of folk medicine. The latest wave of newcomers came from eastern and southern Europe, often from villages and small towns devoid of professional medical care. The absence of doctors and nurses in their isolated European communities forced them to rely on family and local healers to diagnose and treat the sick. In their new homes in Pennsylvania's coal region, racial prejudice and poverty, along with their own cultural preferences, continued immigrants' reliance on both German powwow doctors and their own folk healers. Women played a powerful role as healers throughout the region whether as caretakers for their families or as healers called on by their communities and paid.[13] Healers did not limit themselves to poultices and plasters, herbals, and assorted other ingredients but also included religion and religious symbolism to heal, or at least comfort, the sick.

Hospitals and the Professional Nurse

While it is tempting to believe that the Golden Age of Bacteriology was responsible for the massive increase in the number of hospitals founded in Pennsylvania between 1866 and 1904, the reality is more complex. The great burst in hospital building began after the conclusion of the Civil War, a conflict that impressed on a generation of physicians, nurses, and citizen-soldiers the great benefits of well-managed hospitals. The tremendous fortunes amassed by a growing number of industrialists found a charitable outlet in the funding of hospitals. Though Philadelphia and Pittsburgh were still the centers of wealth in the state, industrial magnates emerged in even very small towns and villages. Thus, while Philadelphia saw a number of important hospitals constructed before 1880, chief among them the Jewish Hospital for the Aged, Infirm and Destitute (now Albert Einstein Hospital) and the Hospital of the University of Pennsylvania (HUP), there was a degree of continuity in the increase of hospitals in the city; Philadelphia was the center of hospital care in the commonwealth before the Civil War, and the city's religious groups, physicians, and wealthy donors continued the trend after the conflict. As such, the history of hospital building in the late nineteenth century beyond the well-heeled confines of Philadelphia is more important to the medical history of Pennsylvania during this period.

Iron production in Pennsylvania rose considerably during the war. Pittsburgh and Allegheny City, the latter annexed as Pittsburgh's Northside in 1905, contained two large arsenals dedicated to producing munitions for the Union. The growing railroads also possessed an insatiable appetite for Pennsylvania-produced iron. Western Pennsylvania, especially Pittsburgh, attracted hundreds of thousands of immigrants, along with thousands more migrants from farms and small towns. In 1865, Pittsburgh boasted three hospitals, a number that grew to five by the end of 1886, when another Catholic Hospital, St. Francis, and the Homeopathic Medical and Surgical Hospital and Dispensary opened. By 1900, ten general hospitals, and several specialized hospitals—for instance, the Eye and Ear Hospital and Children's Hospital—cared for the city's injured and ill.[14]

As astonishing as Pittsburgh's increase in hospitals and hospital beds was after 1865, its hospitals faced increased pressure throughout the late nineteenth century to treat a population that not only grew relentlessly but also experienced injuries and infectious disease on a scale unprecedented in American history as a result of abysmal employment and living conditions.[15] It was not until 1913 that the city outlawed, and began the first weak efforts to eradicate, windowless cellar apartments of the kind New York and Philadelphia abandoned as unfit for habitation during the late nineteenth century.[16] By the late nineteenth century, men like Andrew Carnegie and Henry Clay Frick transformed Pittsburgh into the world's center for iron and steel production.

The steel industry's great wealth came at the cost of an atmosphere burdened with dust from coal fires, blast furnaces, and coke ovens. The pollution produced deaths from pulmonary conditions that soared well above the national average for large industrial cities and became worse over time.[17] Pittsburgh's water supply was even more dangerous than its air. The Allegheny River, which merges with the Monongahela River to form the Ohio River, surged with the waste of 350,000 people by the 1880s, while on the Monongahela sewage barges dumped the contents of the city's cesspits into the river. The rivers were the major source of water for Pittsburgh and dozens of mill towns that lined their banks. Despite Pittsburgh's dangerous environment, the city continued to ignore the need for the sort of large public hospital that Philadelphia had as part of its almshouse complex. The general hospitals of Pittsburgh offered modern surgical and medical services for those who could afford it, but they conducted little research and operated without the benefit of a prominent medical school.

Hospitals had a pronounced effect on the health of people in Pennsylvania's small cities and large towns. Hospitals that opened in small communities began immediately to improve the quality of life. Trauma victims who required, for instance, bone-setting, surgery, removal of foreign objects, or amputation could be treated in a controlled setting, a setting that became cleaner as antiseptic methods continued to be refined. Surgery in a hospital, as opposed to a home or doctor's office, was more likely to be conducted by a surgeon who possessed more training than a town doctor. Recovery, too, was more easily monitored by physicians in a clinical setting, an important factor when one considers the conditions in which many laborers and farmers lived in late nineteenth-century Pennsylvania. Hospitals attracted physicians and nurses to communities and acted as a point of civic pride, a signal that a town had reached a certain level of maturity and civic-mindedness. Towns that played host to large industrial works were guaranteed a surplus of serious injuries, and without a hospital, injured workers could turn only to company infirmaries and local physicians.

A good example of a hospital's effect on an industrial community is provided by St. Luke's Hospital in Fountain Hill. Founded in 1873 and located on the grounds of the defunct Bethlehem Water Cure, St. Luke's received a major infusion of cash in 1879 when industrialist Asa Packer bequeathed $300,000 to the institution.[18] St. Luke's campus was perched on the edge of Lehigh County, about five miles west of Allentown, the county seat. From its location St. Luke's overlooked the South Bethlehem, Northampton County, works of the Bethlehem Iron Company, later Bethlehem Steel Corporation, one of the largest producers of iron and steel in the world. The hospital treated a ceaseless stream of people maimed and burned at the mill, while it cared for another patient pool that emerged from the dilapidated housing and poor sanitation in the workers' neighborhoods. St. Luke's proximity to New York granted the hospital access to physicians in major hospitals, and it managed to acquire the services of William Estes, a surgeon from Mount Sinai Hospital in New York, as its director. Allentown's seriously ill and injured also sought attention at St. Luke's, though their wagon ride over rough roads must have been agonizing. When Allentown founded its first hospital in 1899, its impact on surgical treatment and the general state of medicine in the city was immediate and it, too, attracted physicians from prestigious medical schools and hospitals, including its longtime director, Dr. C. D. Schaeffer, a graduate of the University of Pennsylvania's medical school.[19]

The proliferation of hospitals in Pennsylvania during the last half of the nineteenth century was intimately tied to a surge of nursing programs throughout the state. Throughout the late eighteenth and nineteenth centuries, the number of women who worked as medical providers declined as the medical profession launched assaults against midwifery and, concomitantly, limited medical school entrance to men. The most important exception to the general trend of excluding women from the medical professions was the Women's Medical College, which, by 1910, was recognized as better than most of the traditional medical schools in the nation. As men pushed women out of healthcare, however, physicians and hospitals began to recognize the vital role of professional nurses. The typical hospital employed no trained nurses; rather, nursing care in hospitals varied from one institution to another, with family members of patients often pressed into service. Patients with no family to care for them in the hospital faced grim prospects as most orderlies and nurses were simply other patients pressed into service, or former

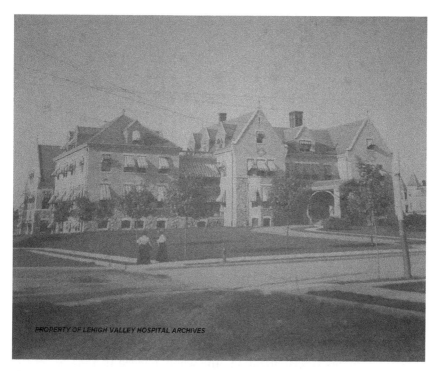

Allentown Hospital, 1899. The hospital opened in 1899 and quickly grew into an important center for specialized care and surgery in an underserved city. Notice the old mansion style of construction. (Courtesy of Lehigh Valley Health Network.)

patients hired by hospitals, but with no training for the job. Basic nursing procedures, such as regular rounds on the ward, supervision of nurses by senior nurses and physicians, and even the basics of wound care and hygiene were almost unknown. In Europe, Florence Nightingale's efforts on behalf of soldiers during the Crimean War of the mid-1850s brought the first widespread attention to the importance of nurses, while America's Clara Barton, a pivotal figure during the Civil War, raised awareness in the United States. Indeed, reformers realized that military, and by extension civilian, hospitals, were only as good as the nursing care such institutions provided patients.

Reformers in Philadelphia moved to implement a higher standard for nurse training and practice as early as 1836, when the Nursing Society of Philadelphia (NSP) was founded in conjunction with a charity dedicated to providing competent obstetric care for poor women.[20] The NSP trained the charity's nurses in best practices for labor and delivery and by 1850 opened a modest school for nursing obstetrics. Obstetric nursing fit nicely into the

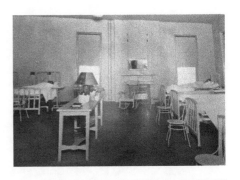

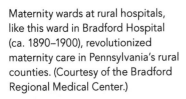

Maternity wards at rural hospitals, like this ward in Bradford Hospital (ca. 1890–1900), revolutionized maternity care in Pennsylvania's rural counties. (Courtesy of the Bradford Regional Medical Center.)

conventional role of women-as-midwives and did not threaten the gender roles that came to define the medical profession by the early nineteenth century. Pennsylvania Hospital inaugurated a nursing school in 1883, while St. Luke's Hospital opened what might be regarded as not only the third nursing school in the state but also the oldest continuously operated nursing school in America, in 1884.[21]

Though the Pennsylvania Hospital and St. Luke's nursing programs were milestones, the nursing school at Philadelphia General Hospital, the city's almshouse, merits special attention. The school opened in 1885 under the direction of two English nurses, Alice Fisher and Edith Horner. Both women had trained under Florence Nightingale and served as senior nurses in major English hospitals, and Fisher remained friends with Nightingale throughout her life. Fisher arrived in Philadelphia in 1883, joined shortly by Horner, who acted as her assistant. Together they formulated plans for the hospital's nursing school and shepherded the school through its first few years, revolutionizing operations at the hospital, which had become increasingly rundown and, in some respects, dangerous to its patients, as orderlies often ran amok, robbing and assaulting their charges. Fisher and Horner established the same procedures in the Philadelphia General Hospital that were used in English institutions. Fisher died in 1888, but her efforts had already produced one of the most respected hospital regimes in the nation, while the school of nursing remained for decades one of the most respected programs in the nation, even when measured against nursing schools opened by prestigious universities and hospitals.

So great was the admiration evinced by Philadelphia nurses for Fisher that, for decades after her death, a procession of nurses from across the city made its way to her grave in solemn remembrance of her achievements. Another noted director of the nursing program, S. Lillian Clayton, graduated from the school of nursing in 1896 and set about directing nursing programs

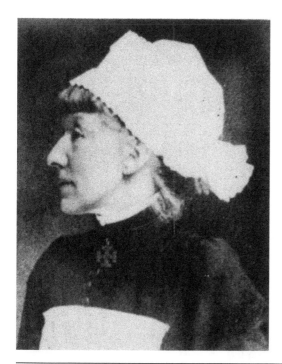

Alice Fisher, ca. 1884–1888. (Courtesy of the Barbara Bates Center for the Study of the History of Nursing.)

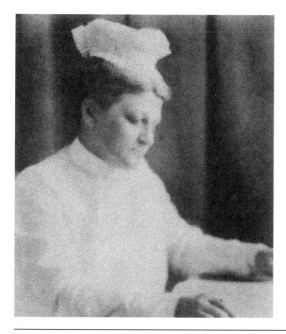

S. Lillian Clayton, ca. 1915–1930. (Courtesy of the Barbara Bates Center for the Study of the History of Nursing.)

in hospitals in Pennsylvania and other states. Clayton assumed the director-ship of the Pennsylvania General Hospital nursing program between 1915 and 1930. One of her chief endeavors was introducing the school's rigorous nursing standards abroad. To this end she accepted large numbers of "foreign students for special courses." Clayton insisted that she wished for "the best in American nursing to be known abroad."[22] Clayton, like Fisher and Horner before her, personified a new archetype of American medical women whose influence moved far beyond the halls of their own hospital and nursing program, and helped shape the contours of modern American healthcare.

As training for nurses in Pennsylvania during the late nineteenth century was almost wholly the preserve of hospitals, not universities, one result of hospital construction, especially in rural areas, was a growing cadre of trained nurses in even the most remote sections of the state.[23] Many of the graduating classes from nurse training programs conducted in small hospitals in towns like Bradford, Lancaster, and Beaver frequently numbered only three or four students. The modest class size belied the power of trained nurses to enhance

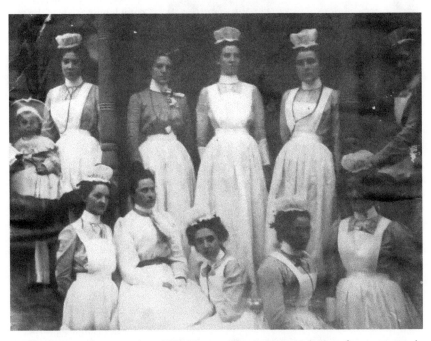

Bradford Hospital nursing class, 1900. The small but important classes of nurses trained and graduated by Bradford Hospital and other rural hospitals provided crucial health services in hospitals and homes throughout the vast expanse of rural Pennsylvania. (Courtesy of the Bradford Regional Medical Center.)

medical services in their communities; nurses served not only in town hospitals but also in doctors' offices, in schools, as visiting nurses, and as an arm of the local and state public health authorities. Nurses were arguably even more valuable in the late nineteenth-century context of medicine than in the context of early twenty-first-century medicine simply because doctors in the late 1800s remained largely powerless to cure disease. Put another way, the Victorian-era physician routinely diagnosed a variety of infectious diseases that modern American doctors rarely see, but unlike modern physicians, late nineteenth-century doctors possessed almost nothing with which to treat infection.

In the face of such impotence, nursing care offered the sole reliable means by which medicine could promote health in the face of infectious disease and a successful recovery after surgery. In an era when there was little precedent for how hospitals should function, nurses like Alice Fisher and Edith Horner brought order out of chaos and ensured patients received regular attention. Nursing, then, provided one of the few spaces in which women might participate in the era's male-dominated medicine, with the ironic twist that they offered more effective treatment than their male physician counterparts. The most important official recognition of the critical role nurses played was a 1909 state law that regulated the education and training of nurses and prohibited anyone from practicing as a nurse without proper licensure.[24]

Public Health

Bacteriology redirected and repositioned public health's role in managing, preventing, and treating disease. By the 1870s, filth was inextricably linked to disease, not because sewage and other filth contained bacteria but because their decomposition and fermentation were understood to produce disease in a way not fully explained by science. Scientists also widely acknowledged that people could transmit illness to others through a mechanism that, like disease allegedly produced by putrefying garbage, was poorly understood. As in earlier eras, cities and towns tried to abate the worst nuisances and enacted minimal standards of rubbish removal, cesspit cleaning, and similar ordinances. Discoveries in the field of bacteriology during the 1880s redirected public health efforts to a focus on isolation and treatment of diseased individuals, all while eliminating sources of contagion in the environment. Public health advocates across Pennsylvania recognized that strong public health bodies, allied to emerging technologies such as water filtration, held the power to transform the health of the entire state.

The Philadelphia board of health remained the most sophisticated and powerful public health organization in the state through the turn of the twentieth century. The board recognized the value of collecting comprehensive vital statistics about its citizens and by the 1870s published annual birth, death, and disease records. The filthiness of Philadelphia's streets, a result not just of crowding but of a corrupt contract system that farmed street cleaning out to private firms with little city oversight, incurred the ire of the board, which took steps in the 1870s to reduce the worst abuses. At the same time, the city discontinued the use of cobblestones as a street-building material, which made street sweeping easier. As for the eternal problem of waste disposal, the board banned the practice of nighttime removal of cesspit material in open carts in favor of daytime removal in sealed tanks that pumped sludge from the cesspit via pipes by the end of the 1870s.[25]

In the 1880s the board of health was reorganized, its governing board reduced from twelve to five, while its cadre of inspectors, engineers, and medical personnel grew. Following a general trend in public health, the board expanded its power throughout the 1880s and 1890s to include food inspection and regulation, especially with regard to the city's milk supply, which was particularly vulnerable to adulteration and spoilage. Compulsory vaccination of school children was also instituted, which, along with milk inspection, decreased rates of childhood mortality. In 1903, the state adopted new legislation that remade the city's board of health into the department of public health and charities and subordinated it to the department of public safety, which included the police and fire departments.

Public medicine in Philadelphia also became more sophisticated during the late 1800s. For instance, the "Old Blockley" hospital, attached to the Philadelphia Almshouse and managed by a board of guardians of the poor rather than by the board of health, not only expanded the hospital's size but also founded a school of nursing on the premises in 1885. The school trained and provided a continuous supply of nurses for the institution to replace the inmates who acted as nurses and orderlies. In the early 1870s, the University of Pennsylvania and its school of medicine moved to a location almost immediately opposite the almshouse and its hospital. The university used the hospital's wards as a training ground for its medical students and physicians. In 1865 Philadelphia opened, under the direction of the board of health, the Municipal Hospital for Contagious Disease, at Twenty-Second and Lehigh Streets.[26] The original intent of the facility was the removal of cases of dangerous infectious disease from Blockley Hospital and the tenements. By the turn of the century, however, the board had the authority to remove all cases of smallpox, anthrax, typhus, and similarly lethal infections to the hospital even if the patients in question possessed the financial resources for treatment in private hospitals.

The sophisticated though overwhelmed public health system in Philadelphia was not mirrored in Pittsburgh. By the 1840s, city politics resulted in the creation of a health warden for each ward. The city did not empower health wardens to correct sanitary problems; rather their role was to record the dimensions of disease outbreaks, count the number of residents in boarding houses, and report to the council and mayor. In 1850, the state passed legislation to create the city's first board of health, which commenced in 1853. The board languished, lapsed, and was reorganized in 1872, did very little work after 1872, and was resurrected and reorganized again in 1888.[27] The mayor appointed the board and such appointments were riven by political intrigue and heavy with men who possessed little understanding of, or experience in, public health.

The public health picture in Pittsburgh was further muddled by an agreement between the state's Republican machine and its counterpart organization in Pittsburgh, the only machine agreement made in writing anywhere in the nation, that allowed the Pittsburgh machine to veto any state health regulations passed by Harrisburg as they pertained to the city, as long as the city's political bosses backed the state machine's candidates and leaders.[28] The appalling environment that confronted Pittsburgh's residents, along with the absence of hospital care for the poor, made the lack of public health efforts especially dangerous. Indeed, observers consider Philadelphia's death rates from infectious disease relatively high, in part because Philadelphia is often compared to New York, whose public health efforts accomplished a great deal even as millions of immigrants crowded its tenements. When Philadelphia is compared to Pittsburgh, however, the City of Brotherly Love seems a monument to sanitation and hygiene.

Beyond the metropolises of Philadelphia and Pittsburgh, in the rural districts, towns, and small cities where most citizens lived, public health standards, nuisance abatement, and anti-epidemic measures were managed according to local resources and prerogatives. Furthermore, no state board of health existed to aid communities in either the planning of effective public health strategies or the fight against disease outbreaks, with the result that rural townships enjoyed virtually no protections from sanitary dangers and could not reliably fight epidemics. The most common model of public health work in such communities was one in which temporary boards were created to manage outbreaks and then disbanded, with all other local laws concerning public health handled as sanitary codes, exactly the sort of public health policy Philadelphia employed more than a century earlier. As late as 1886, of the 574 municipalities in Pennsylvania, only 11 maintained permanent health boards.[29]

State Board of Health

Massachusetts was the first state to create a statewide board of health in 1869, followed by two dozen other states by the mid-1880s. The power of a state board to help its citizens was largely determined by the legislative parameters that lawmakers constructed and within which any state board operated. At a minimum a state board acted in an advisory role by suggesting to the legislature ways to improve a host of health-related conditions in the state. In rural areas that lacked a town or county board, a state board acted as the primary responder to outbreaks and other public health emergencies. Some state boards were also empowered to regulate threats to the public health, extending the same protections to rural areas that citizens of municipalities with enough resources, and the political will, to adopt health legislation and boards of their own enjoyed. Pennsylvania, especially when one considers its wealth and the extent of its medical establishment, faced a long and difficult battle to found a state board.

As science increasingly recognized that some diseases were contagious, and the germ theory of disease spread through the ranks of Pennsylvania's medical establishment, the medical society of Pennsylvania began to push for a state board of health. A state board, the society argued in a familiar vein, would cover those areas of the state with few medical resources, and with proper authority a state board could not only respond to epidemics but also prevent them by enacting minimum sanitary standards.[30] As a corollary to a state board, the society also believed that the state should collect the vital statistics of its residents in an effort to gauge threats to health. Three attempts to pass a bill independent of any input by the society failed between 1872 and 1874. In 1875, the society took up the cause and began a lobbying campaign in Harrisburg, as well as a publicity campaign in newspapers and professional conferences, that spanned the next decade.

Lack of political will in Harrisburg certainly helped stymie passage of a bill, but so did antipathy, and even hostility, on the part of many in the public. One of the chief concerns was that tax money would be flung once again into the maw of another corrupt bureau composed of political appointees. A newspaper in Norristown saw a state board of health as nothing more than yet another expensive boondoggle and suggested that "it was a pretty safe rule to discourage all legislation having for its object the creating of additional public offices."[31] The editor of a Harrisburg newspaper cast doubt on the validity of arguments advanced by reformers that the board would serve on a voluntary basis by arguing that "they, while pretending to serve for nothing, will run up a bill of expenses which in comparison to services rendered will be about as a mountain to a mole hill."[32]

Financial concerns were not the only objections raised against a state board of health. Professional animosity between the allopathic medical community and unconventional practitioners, especially homeopaths, also contributed to the repeated rejection of bills to create a board of health. This was especially the case when the Pennsylvania Medical Society began to champion the creation of a state board as part of its mission. The society believed that a board should be composed of only members of the allopathic medical profession. For their part, homeopaths, whose political power was considerable, feared that without a seat on a board of health, a state board could be used as a weapon by allopaths to bludgeon homeopathic medicine into extinction through the construction and imposition of licensing requirements that recognized only their allopathic counterparts as "real" medicine. Such a board, especially if granted regulatory authority, might legislate homeopathy out of existence in Pennsylvania, or at least curtail the power of unconventional medicine to the extent that it lost any real power to treat its patients as it saw fit. For the homeopathic community, then, the fight against a state board that did not allow for a homeopathic voice translated into a fight for the very survival of their discipline.[33]

The most vocal of the reformers was Benjamin Lee, a pioneering orthopedic physician from Philadelphia who evinced a decades-long commitment to public health and the construction of a state board of health. Lee was a prominent member of the state medical society and used his connections in both that society and the public health circles of Philadelphia to advocate for a state board of health. Lee, a devout Christian, often paired his passion for the public good with his own interpretation of the Bible to argue for sanitation and hygiene as endeavors that not only served the needs of humanity but also honored the Almighty. In one of his most forceful addresses, he suggested that "physicians, jurists, divines, editors" had a duty to influence legislators so that the state would join "the sisterhood of intelligent and progressive commonwealths who possess a State Board of Health."[34] Yet even the efforts of Benjamin Lee could not move the legislature to act; what was required was an epidemic to highlight Pennsylvania's utter inability to assist its citizens during an outbreak.

In 1885 the town of Plymouth, Luzerne County, with a population of about eight thousand, lay perched on the side of several steep mountains, the bottom reaches of the hamlet along the west bank of the Susquehanna River, a few miles outside Wilkes-Barre. It is difficult to imagine that anything that happened in such an obscure town possessed the power to shatter the political inertia in Harrisburg that had for years blocked every effort to construct a state board. Today, the slopes of the mountains above Plymouth are covered by forest, but by the mid-1880s coal mining, and the breakers that smashed the coal into usable pieces while leaving piles of slag, had long since denuded the mountains of trees. The ugly scars of bare rock overlay ground that sank and shifted as the mines that cut into the mountains collapsed and killed miners, and were just as quickly replaced by new mines, new miners, and new disasters. Several small streams emerged from the same rock holding the coal that built the wealth of some even as it condemned most of the town's people to a hellish existence. Streams careened down the mountains following the ravines that separate one mountain from another, the water clear and sweet until, passing near the mines, they were loaded with acidic mine drainage.

One of those insignificant streams, whose name was never recorded in contemporary newspaper accounts, official state reports, or by the numerous historians who highlighted the events in Plymouth, was named Coal Creek, just as locals refer to it in the early twenty-first century. Coal Creek begins its journey at a spring at the top of Shawnee Mountain and courses about three miles from its source to the town. In the mid-1870s, investors formed the Plymouth Water Company and decided to use the cold, clear water as their main source of supply for the town. The water company constructed four dams in relatively level areas along Coal Creek's run and thereby created four small reservoirs, which locals and records sometimes termed ponds.[35] The company also installed an eight-inch cast-iron pipe that delivered a continuous supply of water to its pumping station. The largest of the reservoirs was the fourth, or topmost, reservoir on the summit of the mountain. By the early 1880s, the family of John Davis built a modest home along Coal Creek between the third and fourth reservoirs, about one hundred feet from the bank of the stream, and operated a small dairy farm whose milk they sold to the residents of Plymouth.

In late 1884, John Davis visited his brother in Philadelphia. His brother lived in a building that experienced several cases of typhoid during Davis's stay. He returned to Plymouth a very sick man in January 1885 and spent the next few months fighting for his life against the ravages of a severe case of typhoid. A nurse who tended Davis threw his bacteria-laden feces on the snow beside the stream during evening hours, and during the day she dumped his excrement into the family's outhouse, where the contents leached into the stream. The spring melt carried the bacteria into the stream and the third collection pond. The first definitive cases of typhoid emerged in April, but it

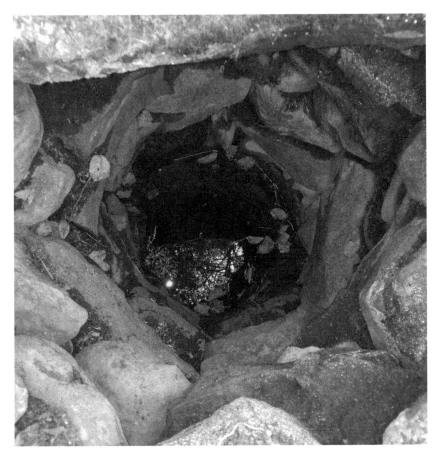

The outhouse hole of the Jones family homestead, 2019. This outhouse hole was responsible for igniting the Plymouth typhoid epidemic that ended with the founding of the state board of health. (Courtesy of James E. Higgins and Aydan Kirby.)

was not until mid-May, after scores had already fallen ill and dozens of deaths occurred, that autopsies confirmed the presence of the disease.[36] The epidemic rapidly overran the meager medical resources in Plymouth while neither the county nor the state possessed the authority or personnel to direct a response. The vacuum was filled by physicians from Wilkes-Barre and Philadelphia who traveled at their own expense to aid the town. When the epidemic subsided at the end of the summer, 114 people were dead and public opinion swung in favor of a state board of health.

The state board of health commenced operations in the spring of 1886, with Benjamin Lee as its secretary for the entire twenty years of its existence. Under its charter, the board was responsible for investigating outbreaks and sanitary dangers but had no mandate to issue violations (the compendium of state laws included no sanitary laws) or power to enact ordinances or standards. As one reformer put it, the board could only educate and study; it could not mandate.[37] The task of collecting the state's vital statistics was far too large for the poorly resourced board, so it instead collected such statistics from local authorities, though most municipalities and townships did not collect such data. The state board of health, then, was generally an inoffensive—and ineffective—state advisory group that arrived during or after an outbreak of infectious disease. Communities stricken by an epidemic could request that the board assume responsibility for fighting an outbreak. At other times, local authorities simply requested the board advise as to best practices in control and treatment. In either case, the state board could do little more than marshal local resources because the state did not equip the board with the authority, equipment, or personnel to carry the fight against an epidemic on its own. The board also recommended preventive measures, including water testing and filtration, to spare communities from future epidemics of typhoid. The board described the condition of the state's water supplies and the sickness and deaths that resulted as "a crime as great, as cruel, and as shameful as the slaughter of the innocents in sacred history."[38] As the nineteenth century entered its final decade, the deficiencies inherent in the legislation that created the board, combined with budget cuts caused by an economic depression, hampered the board's effectiveness in even its very limited role.

By the turn of the twentieth century, reformers in the ranks of Pennsylvania medicine spearheaded an effort to replace the state's moribund board of health with a robust department of health headed by a cabinet-level commissioner. If Benjamin Lee midwifed the birth of the board of health, then Charles Penrose was most responsible for ushering the department of health into being. Penrose belonged to a powerful Philadelphia family, and his brother Boies was a powerful leader in the state Republican machine and a United States senator.[39] Charles Penrose earned his medical degree at Harvard, practiced in Philadelphia, and became a noted gynecologist. By the early twentieth century, Penrose conceived of legislation to found a strong department of health and, importantly, his brother Boies pledged not to turn the department into a patronage machine. Even with the acquiescence of Boies, the legislature refused to consider a bill. As in the struggle for the board of health, the rights of property owners, budgetary concerns, and corporate interests opposed the legislation. An additional anxiety was a fear that an intrusive department of health smacked of socialism.

As was the case with authorizing the board of health, the legislature was prompted to take more action by an epidemic of typhoid, this time in the western Pennsylvania mill town of Butler. Butler's thirteen thousand residents relied on filtered water supplied by a private company. In August 1903 a small dam broke and contaminated the drinking supply, and the water company kept this news, and the fact that it temporarily switched off its filtration equipment to clean its small reservoir, from the community. The first few cases of typhoid emerged in early autumn and by November ballooned into more than 400 cases. The epidemic did not cease until January, after it killed 111, sickened 1,348, and virtually halted Butler's economy.[40] The state board of health sent a bacteriologist to confirm the nature of the disease, while another physician sent on the board's behalf advised Butler's health board on prevention of typhoid and treatment. Though twenty years had passed since the Plymouth typhoid epidemic, the state remained almost powerless to take decisive action in the event of an outbreak. The commonwealth's inability to aid its citizens shocked Pennsylvanians. Furthermore, the plight of Butler's residents, as well as the shoddy nature of Pennsylvania's public health infrastructure and the poor quality of many of the state's municipal water supplies, generated a great deal of publicity—and embarrassment—in the national press.

The combination of reformers' pressure on the state to construct a credible state health department, and the bad publicity shined on the state's quality of health, precipitated a push in the legislature and the governor's office for passage of a comprehensive package of laws to establish a cabinet-level department of health with authority to regulate and eliminate sanitary dangers, respond to epidemics, collect vital statistics, and clean up Pennsylvania's streams. Much of the language in the bill was written by Charles Penrose, though he declined to act as the department's leader.[41] The broad powers proposed for the department required Governor Samuel Pennypacker to select a commissioner who would avoid the temptation to unduly interfere in business operations or the rights of property owners, yet produce results commensurate with the wishes of health reformers and a citizenry that was increasingly inclined to accept progressive solutions to society's problems.[42] Pennypacker settled on Samuel Gibson Dixon, a lawyer and physician who earned his degrees at the University of Pennsylvania. Dixon had already studied with several of Europe's most prominent scientists and physicians, opened the hygiene laboratory at University of Pennsylvania, made important discoveries with regard to the tuberculosis bacterium, and gone on to assume the presidency of the Academy of Natural Sciences of Philadelphia.

Before he accepted his appointment, Dixon insisted he be allowed to continue as president of the Academy of Natural Sciences, a position he kept until his death concluded his time as both commissioner of health and president of the academy. Dixon also demanded that he alone be allowed to select personnel for the department of health, free from political interference and intrigue. The governor agreed that politicizing the department would only undermine its position. With these guarantees in place, and legislation that granted his department of health more power than the health department of any other state, Pennsylvania freed Dixon to actualize a plan for transforming the state's health that he had begun to formulate more than a decade earlier. At the core of his blueprint for a markedly healthier commonwealth was a powerful, science-driven department whose purview was the entire state. Dixon, his methods always rooted in firm empirical ground, nevertheless managed to avoid inflaming political or industry sensibilities and thereby ensured his department received accolades and funding.

Conclusion

The years 1866–1905 encompassed the most dynamic period in the history of Pennsylvania medicine. Discoveries in European laboratories, and the new paradigm of disease causation, prevention, and treatment they spawned, swept over Pennsylvania. The most pronounced effects were felt in Philadelphia because its universities, medical schools, and physicians controlled the most, and certainly the best, medical resources in the commonwealth. Beyond Philadelphia, the new knowledge brushed aside prior concepts to such a degree that by 1900 few physicians in even the most remote portions of the state believed in any concept of infectious disease other than the germ theory. Hospitals and nurses, both of which benefited from new antiseptic techniques and sanitary precautions, preserved the lives of people who would otherwise have died. Most importantly, in terms of Pennsylvania's commitment to the health and welfare of its citizens, reformers fought and won a battle for a state board of health, and when the board failed to realize the goals reformers set, a department of health was brought into being.

The advances in Pennsylvania's medical and public health infrastructures were not simply the result of new technology; they also required the political will of legislators and governors, the interest and input of physicians, and the support and submission of the commonwealth's people. The delay in building a proper state department of health cost an unknown number, but certainly thousands, of Pennsylvanians their lives. The next period of Pennsylvania's history witnessed the state's department of health remake the health of the state's people, especially rural folk, while Pittsburgh's health fell ever further behind other large cities in the nation. Despite the inroads made against bacterial infections, Pennsylvania medicine stood seemingly powerless when the deadliest epidemic in history ravaged the state during the closing months of World War I. Yet such loss too often overshadowed the increasingly powerful role Pennsylvania played in helping chart the course of medicine and health during the first decades of the twentieth century.

4

TRIUMPHS AND TRIBULATIONS OF
PUBLIC HEALTH, 1906–1945

B Y 1906, PENNSYLVANIA POSSESSED most of the components necessary
to offer middle-class citizens a standard of medical care not imagined
even two decades earlier. The state's rural and urban poor benefited
from advances in sanitation and healthcare, but distribution of resources and
quality of care was uneven and handicapped by the lack of state oversight.
Medical education received a boost to its quality when the Flexner Report
surveyed every degree-granting medical school in the nation and offered rec-
ommendations intended to strengthen the programs of existent schools and
identify those that warranted closure.

As the public health and medical apparatus of the state rapidly improved, America's entry into World War I placed incredible stress on every
aspect of the state's infrastructure, especially medicine and public health.
In the midst of the war, in cities and coal patches packed with war workers,
the worst pandemic in history descended on Pennsylvania and its belea-
guered corps of healthcare workers. Later, the curtailed budgets of Pennsylvania's citizens as well as its state and local governments during the Great
Depression placed new demands on public health, even as war clouds gathered in Europe and Asia. By the end of 1945, the state lay poised to relinquish its involvement in most aspects of public healthcare delivery as private medicine, aided by new drugs and other technological innovations,
assumed increased control of the health and medicine of Pennsylvania's
citizens.

The Hex Murder(s)

By the close of the 1920s, modernity had remade much of Pennsylvania. Its cities and large towns glowed at night, lit by the innumerable electric lights that less than a generation before replaced the flicker of gas lamps. The telephone, a novelty as late as World War I, was becoming a common feature of the middle-class home, while the horse virtually disappeared as a mode of personal transportation. Society granted women the right to vote at almost the same time it stripped anyone of the right to drink alcohol. In the heart of rural Pennsylvania, however, the imprint of the modern age was far more modest. Large swaths of farmland remained unmechanized, with plows still pulled by horses and water drawn by hand from wells more than a century old. In the most remote regions of Pennsylvania Dutch country, modern medicine still shared space with the powwow healer, the power of the germ theory sometimes overruled by belief in the hex.

During the late nineteenth century, the hex or powwow doctor was increasingly viewed as an anachronistic remnant of Pennsylvania's prescientific, rural past. Though the powwowers and their patients might be viewed by their educated, often urbanized neighbors as foolish, only rarely did commentators label the practice dangerous. As the twentieth century dawned, however, powwowing increasingly came to be seen as an insidious, sometimes cultish presence in the otherwise bucolic farmland of Lancaster, York, and Berks counties. Powwow doctors found themselves referred to in the local press as witches, or as hex doctors for the negative association of the term with witches and curses. One newspaper noted that the city of "Reading would be a rare field for the student in psychology now. The only reason she is not burning witches is because the law won't let her."[1] Conventional medicine provided much of the impetus for the hostility. Physicians and coroners throughout the Dutch counties related experiences with people who relied not on orthodox physicians but on powwowers, with death or grievous injury the result. This was especially true in the case of children whose parents, often painted as ignorant wretches, summoned the local hex doctor to treat children with a bag of charms and some prayers, with fatal results.[2]

After decades of decline, powwowing suffered its worst blow not from allopathic medicine but at the hands of three men who believed fervently in powwow's potential to cure disease and banish hexes. About ten miles outside the town of Red Lion, York County, a major stop on the railway and a town that possessed all the trappings of technology the 1920s offered, was the home of Nelson Rehmeyer, a sixty-year-old farmer. People in the area believed that Rehmeyer was a powerful powwow doctor.[3] One of those who believed in Rehmeyer's power was John Blymyer, a thirty-year-old farm laborer who spent time in a state hospital for the insane and on one occasion escaped from the institution. After his release, Blymyer continued to suffer from night sweats, felt generally unwell, and appeared thin. In the midst of these and other physical complaints, Blymyer noticed that his pigs, hitherto healthy and fat, had begun to die. One of Blymyer's neighbors was eighteen-year-old Wilbert Hess. The young man's parents also owned a farm beset with problems, including the closing of one of the roads that serviced the farm and the deaths of a number of chickens.[4]

Blymyer was convinced that his misfortunes and those of the Hess family were the result not of bad luck but of something more sinister. He sought the advice of a woman in the nearby town of Marietta, along the Susquehanna River. The woman, named Emma Knopp, but better known as Nellie Noll, had yet another moniker, River Witch. Blymyer related to Knopp his ills and those of the Hess family, which she pronounced the work of a hex cast by Rehmeyer. To lift the hex, Knopp directed Blymyer to obtain a lock of Rehmeyer's hair as well as his book of incantations and rituals. The hair and book should be either burned or buried—records mention both means of disposal—after which the hex would be lifted.

On the night of November 27, 1928, Blymyer, Hess, and a fourteen-year-old boy named John Curry, who went along because he believed it all a great adventure, entered Rehmeyer's home and demanded his book of spells. When Rehmeyer refused to relinquish either his hair or his book, the trio attacked him, an assault the robust, six-foot-tall Rehmeyer managed to fend off until his assailants slipped a rope around his neck and strangled him while young Curry beat him over the head with a piece of wood. After he fell to the floor dead, the men tried to set his body afire to destroy evidence of their crime, but their attempt at arson failed, and the body was discovered by a neighbor a couple of days later. The investigation aroused renewed interest in powwowing among the public and caused deep consternation among the many Pennsylvania Germans who viewed powwowing as a kind of black magic, not a healing art.

Reports about the "county's latest witchcraft sacrifice" also alluded to at least one other death, that of sixteen-year-old Gertrude Rudy only a year before, as possibly linked "to the operation of witch doctors connected to the Rehmeyer case."[5] Furthermore, links between the killers and other powwowers/witch doctors, including Emma Knopp, were cited as reasons for an official investigation that authorities hoped would stamp out "the operations of the cult."[6] The three killers, tried and convicted of murder, were all eventually released from prison after decades behind bars, and all of the men appear to have led normal lives until they died during the 1960s and 1970s. The spotlight the case put on both powwowing and Pennsylvania Dutch culture as backward and even dangerous changed the contours of powwowing forever. Over the next few years, authorities suspected that several deaths in Berks and Northampton Counties were tied to powwow/hex rituals, though very little evidence was ever produced to validate such claims.

Though it never entirely disappeared, powwow is regarded as an antique folkway by most people, even among rural Pennsylvania Dutch. Nevertheless, even in the early twenty-first century, powwowers and witches hold powerful sway over some. For instance, the owners of the homestead of Marie Jung found that they had to cajole a local stonemason, an older Pennsylvania Dutch man, into repairing the low stone wall around the grave of the Jung family.[7] The stonemason put the owners off for months because he feared Mountain Mary's power. In Marietta, a staff member in borough hall recalled that while she and her siblings were growing up in the 1960s, her parents threatened that the River Witch would get them if they misbehaved.[8] Her parents, children in the 1940s, remembered seeing Nellie Noll, as they knew her, stand on the balcony of the home where she lived. Similarly, the owner of a tavern down the street from Noll's home remembered that, as a boy in the 1960s, he bagged Noll's groceries in a local supermarket. She had long white hair, would not speak even when he tried to converse with her, and generally appeared like the personification of a "witch," though he thought it more likely that she was simply a lonely, elderly woman with few friends and a reclusive lifestyle.[9]

Academic Medicine

The quality of medical education and research conducted in Pennsylvania's universities improved markedly in the early twentieth century. This was in part a result of the maturation of European techniques in the hands of American scientists. While the late nineteenth century saw the founding and expansion of medical schools and laboratories in Pennsylvania, and better-trained physicians were emerging as early as the 1880s from some of the state's universities, it was the early twentieth century that saw a wave of research and discoveries, the result of an entire generation of scientifically proficient medical minds coupled with well-equipped labs. Research and medical education in Pennsylvania continued to concentrate in Philadelphia, but Pittsburgh's medical institutions grew more robust at the dawn of the twentieth century, too.

When Temple University's medical school opened in 1901, it required five years of part-time education beyond high school, a higher standard than most medical programs in the country. Within a few years, the university was renowned for its hands-on approach to medical education. The initial response of the city's elite physicians, that Temple might offer an inferior degree to an inferior student body, not only reflected racial and religious prejudices but also highlighted the pride of place and the sensitivity of Philadelphia's medical community to the excellence of the city's medical schools. The care with which a medical education in Philadelphia was treated by the profession was reflected in a seminal study in the early twentieth century.

In 1910, the Carnegie Foundation released the Flexner Report, a survey of all 155 schools that offered medical degrees in America and Canada. Most of the schools offered a two-year program with little laboratory or clinical training, and even the best schools rarely demanded students have anything beyond a high school diploma. The report characterized many schools in the nation as shameful, and remarked that some could produce "no justification for their existence."[10] The medical schools of Philadelphia, however, generally received high marks, with the University of Pennsylvania and Jefferson in the top ranks.[11] Western Pennsylvania's only medical school, the University of Pittsburgh, earned a passing grade, but also received high praise for "a complete transformation" of its course of study and faculty in the twelve months prior to the Flexner study.[12] The first step in the transformation included recruiting the best talent available for its corps of professors. Chief among the new faculty was Oscar Klotz, a brilliant thirty-three-year-old pathologist from McGill University who had already proved the role of high blood pressure in arteriosclerosis.[13] Another prominent member of the faculty was William Watt Graham Maclachlan, a noted pneumonia expert whose field studies profited from the dreadful rates of pneumonia in Pittsburgh and who, like Klotz, went on to publish dozens of important papers in his field.

One of the many benefits of the improved level of medical education in the state was a significant increase in research output. One indispensable tool for research remains a line of rats bred by the Wistar Institute of Philadelphia. The Wistar Institute bred the world's first specialized laboratory rat in 1906, and according to some estimates, fully half of all lab rats today are related to the Wistar line.[14] At the Municipal Hospital for Contagious Disease, B. Franklin Royer, a graduate of Jefferson Medical College with a remarkable knack for scientific investigation, used his new position as the hospital's chief physician to establish a laboratory for the immediate assay of specimens.[15] Royer's ulterior motive was his conviction that a contagious disease hospital in a city as large as Philadelphia offered unparalleled opportunities to explore disease pathology and treatment. After experimenting with different dosages of diphtheria antitoxin, as well as prophylactic doses for family members and others in close contact with diphtheria cases, Royer concluded that several high doses of antitoxin yielded better results than the then-standard smaller doses.[16] He also recommended that physicians use antitoxin in all suspected cases of diphtheria even before laboratory analysis of sputum confirmed the diagnosis. Royer's suggestions quickly became a best practice throughout the nation's hospitals.

Other important research focused on pneumonia, a pernicious disease throughout the country but one to which Pennsylvanians proved especially vulnerable largely because of the commonwealth's lung-damaging industrial jobs. Coal miners in both the eastern anthracite and western bituminous fields suffered from a variety of lung diseases caused by inhalation of mineral dust. The state's many iron and steel workers, as well as laborers in coke works, also inhaled rock dust by virtue of their proximity to combusted coal and smelting furnaces. In addition to work-related hazards, workers and their families suffered from poor diets and terrible living conditions. These factors produced high mortality rates from pneumonia. The first large, systematic study of the disease began in Philadelphia in February 1916 under the auspices of the Phipps Institute and the city department of health. The study noted links between living conditions and mortality rates, as well as comprehensive bacteriological breakdowns of dozens of cases. Additionally, the study suggested that the twenty-five thousand African Americans who hailed from the South, mostly from rural areas, were not accustomed to either urban living conditions or the cold winter months and therefore developed "pneumonia of a virulent type."[17] Such a declaration may have carried racial overtones, of course, yet the army, too, noted in studies of its troops that contingents of rural soldiers who mixed with soldiers from cities always suffered higher rates of death from respiratory disease than their urban comrades. The Philadelphia pneumonia study was cited hundreds of times by scholars over the next decade.

Medical care in early to mid-twentieth-century Pennsylvania defies generalization. In 1910, a middle-class family in Philadelphia had access to a family doctor trained in germ theory, receptive to antitoxin and vaccination, well versed in isolation of infectious disease cases, and practicing in one of the nation's medical centers with ready access to hospitals in cases of trauma or for operations. By 1910 aspirin was readily available, a sort of miracle drug that reduced fever, pain, and inflammation with few of the side effects caused by other drugs used for those symptoms. Yet family doctors, about whom lies the warm glow of nostalgia, found themselves almost powerless against common bacterial diseases until the 1930s and the introduction of sulfon-amides, though the introduction of penicillin and other antibiotics after World War II had the greatest impact on bacterial infections. Indeed, what are now viewed as "ordinary" sore throats, bronchitis, and pneumonia did not yield to even the most skilled physician and often developed into serious ill-ness and ended in death. In contrast to a middle-class urban family, a pros-perous farming family—members of Pennsylvania's agricultural gentry—faced different medical realities. For instance, though most physicians accepted the germ theory by 1910, rural areas often neglected antitoxin and vaccination, with the result that people died needlessly. The patient's home or doctor's office were the preferred sites for operations, and nursing care was often thin. Cases of serious trauma took hours to remove to hospitals in ad-jacent counties, and many died in transit.

In the early twenty-first century, seeking care from a specialist is a regu-lar, even anticipated, part of healthcare. For most of Pennsylvania's history, however, patients rarely encountered the trained specialist. Hospitals facili-tated the growth of specialized medical care because they could afford to support doctors who did not practice primary or surgical care, or practiced it in addition to their narrow field of expertise. In some sense, hospitals during the late nineteenth century were partly successful because they drew together physicians, surgeons, roentgenologists, and obstetricians, among others, in a continuously expanding list of specialty fields. But the specialist as a private practice physician came of age in the decades before World War II. Special-ization occurred first in large urban areas and, when the economies of smaller communities could sustain such services, specialist practices expanded to fill the niche.[18] Though subtly at first, specialist practices inexorably whittled away at the expectations placed on family doctors by their patients.

Public Heath

The 1905 founding of the state department of health appeared to promise citizens an improved quality of life by means of a vigorous program of state-sponsored public health measures made effective through the creation and enforcement of a comprehensive body of laws. In 1886, the state board of health, also envisioned by reformers as a transformative public health force, fell far short of its champions' goals. The new department faced the same entrenched interests committed to hobbling the department and its leader, Samuel G. Dixon. Unlike the board of health, however, the department prof-ited from a shift in attitude among Pennsylvanians with respect to political and social problems. The period from roughly 1900 until the conclusion of

World War I constituted the bulk of the period known as the Progressive Era, when middle-class reformers used a mixture of technology, legislation, and education to effect change in many areas of life. For the department of health, progressives provided the political will that allowed the department to act even when powerful interests were arrayed against it. The Progressive Era notwithstanding, health reformers had begun to agitate a quarter century earlier, in the 1870s, for stronger measures to ensure the public's health both at the state and local levels and might be fairly regarded as among the state's earliest modern reformers in a progressive vein.

Armed with a budget of almost $200,000 for 1906 (more than $5 million in today's money), Dixon spent his first year identifying and hiring the top public health talent, divided the state into ten health districts, and hired two hundred health officers and sanitary inspectors. The danger of tuberculosis compelled the legislature to place responsibility for tuberculosis control in the hands of the department of health, and Dixon opened dozens of dispensaries and several large tuberculosis sanitaria in the state for long-term treatment of tuberculosis cases. The state's network of tuberculosis hospitals and clinics was augmented by a growing corps of state tuberculosis nurses who visited the ill at home and staffed the clinics and hospitals. Between 1907 and 1914, the state's nurses and physicians examined and treated more than one hundred thousand patients and their family members. The department was also tasked with devising a system to collect the state's vital statistics, a goal that the old board of health found so elusive over the course of its twenty-year existence. Dixon mandated reporting of births, marriages, and cause of death by physicians, midwives, and local government bodies. So complete were the state's statistics that the census bureau immediately included the state in the federal registration area and adopted some of Dixon's methods of statistical compilation.[19]

Rural communities felt the power of the new department well before the state's cities because the department was often the sole public health body, and often the only real medical care available. Antitoxins for diphtheria and tetanus, for instance, were not available in wide swaths of the state until Dixon made the department responsible for distributing it to the ill through either local doctors or state-run dispensaries.[20] Rural water supplies, which often dated to ponds and wells excavated during the colonial era, became increasingly dangerous as the rural population grew and human and industrial waste reached the water table or went directly into surface waters. Dixon's men, especially B. Franklin Royer, whom Dixon appointed as the state's chief medical inspector in 1910, spent much of their time ordering the cleanup of township water supplies and the redressing of other hazards to

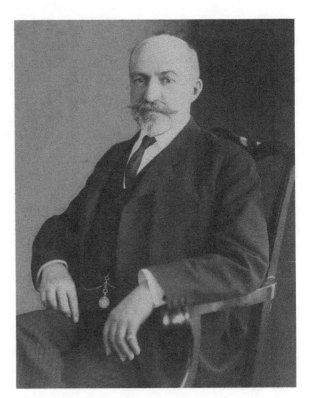

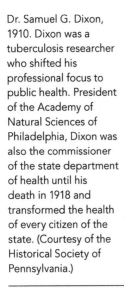

Dr. Samuel G. Dixon, 1910. Dixon was a tuberculosis researcher who shifted his professional focus to public health. President of the Academy of Natural Sciences of Philadelphia, Dixon was also the commissioner of the state department of health until his death in 1918 and transformed the health of every citizen of the state. (Courtesy of the Historical Society of Pennsylvania.)

health. The power of the department extended only very weakly to Philadelphia and Pittsburgh.

After all, both cities were not only large but also politically powerful and had for decades run their own affairs with regard to public health. Nevertheless, the benefits of the department to the people of Pennsylvania between 1906 and 1917, the last full year of Dixon's stewardship, were immense. The state managed to reduce its typhoid death rate from 56.5 per 100,000 in 1906 to 23.9 per 100,000 in 1909, a drop that saved roughly 2,363 lives.[21] By 1917, the department of health claimed to have preserved up to 120,266 lives.[22] In fairness, the state department of health cannot be credited with the entire drop in mortality rates from infectious disease as several had already begun a slow decline in the state, especially diphtheria and tuberculosis, though the department's efforts accelerated the decline in fatalities. As well, improvements in the water supplies in Philadelphia and Pittsburgh contributed to the overall decline in infant mortality and mortality from typhoid and other waterborne illnesses.

An important counterpoint to the success of the state department of health and the efforts on the part of the Philadelphia department of health was the board of health of Pittsburgh. A weak organization, Pittsburgh's board confined itself mostly to the inspection of restaurants and the milk supply, as well as ineffective monitoring of housing, its deficiencies in this regard highlighted by the awful nature of the city's tenements. The one significant positive development in the city's public health, the implementation of water filtration in 1908 after more than a dozen years of political bickering, had nothing to do with the board. City authorities knew by the late 1880s that typhoid bacteria contaminated most of the city's wells as well as the rivers from which residents drank.

The city commissioned a study group in 1896 to examine water filtration methods in anticipation of a bond issue, but machine bosses, who publicly feared a rise in taxes, and privately squabbled over the awarding of contracts, delayed the building and opening of the filtration works for more than a decade.[23] During the first year of its operation, deaths from typhoid in Pittsburgh dropped from a nation-leading 130 per 100,000 to a rate consistent with the national average for large cities.[24] Between deaths from typhoid, dysentery, and other waterborne diseases, the dozen-year delay cost as many as a thousand lives a year between 1897 and 1908, a pitiful example of politics delaying implementation of available, reliable sanitary technology.

World War I

The opening of hostilities in Europe in July 1914 immediately affected Pennsylvania because of its heavy concentration of ferrous metals industries, coal mines, and large pool of potential laborers with specialized industrial skills. Just months after the war commenced, the Westinghouse manufacturing firm in Pittsburgh received an order for three million shells from the British military.[25] Long before America entered the war in April 1917, a wartime shift in the state's population caused a migration into urban areas throughout the state. The phenomenon touched even the smallest steel mill towns and coal villages. One of the consequences was an increase in the density of population in urban dwellings and a consequent reduction of sanitary and hygiene standards. The official census estimate of Philadelphia's population in 1918 was 1.7 million, but some scholars estimate the population as closer to 2 million.[26] Workers labored six or seven days per week, and housing was at such a premium that some men and women slept on mattresses rented in eight-hour increments to three shifts of boarders.[27]

The crowding of people in filthy living conditions propagated the spread of seemingly every sort of germ ever encountered in Pennsylvania with the exception of yellow fever and cholera. In Philadelphia, rates of mumps, measles, pneumonia, influenza, and meningitis climbed to heights not seen for more than a decade, and prompted the Phipps Institute to ally itself with the city department of health to study the situation and best practices for treatment.[28] In Pittsburgh, the wartime migration sparked not only a rise in every infectious disease category but an outbreak of smallpox among African Americans in the Hill District, too.[29] In fact, conditions for African American migrants in the city were even worse than the conditions that very poor European immigrants faced. For instance, pneumonia deaths increased by 200 percent among African Americans between 1915 and 1917, while deaths outnumbered births in the African American community by 50 percent.[30]

Polio, too, made its first widespread appearance in Philadelphia in the summer of 1916, and from there spread to Pittsburgh, Wilkes-Barre, Lancaster, and a few other large towns, until almost 2,200 cases were officially reported.[31] In light of a modern understanding of polio virus, thousands of others were infected but not diagnosed or tallied because polio is usually a mild illness that did not warrant a trip to the doctor. Philadelphia not only accounted for most cases of polio in the state but also had more than two hundred deaths from the disease during the summer and autumn. The deaths, combined with the fact that that most of the dead and paralyzed were children, frightened every parent with young children in the city.[32]

The following year, Pennsylvania's medical community heeded America's call to arms with an enthusiasm difficult to imagine. Even before America declared war, hospitals across the state organized themselves along the lines of military field hospital units complete with uniforms and equipment. By 1917, for instance, so many of the physicians and professors of the University of Pittsburgh's medical school had already volunteered and done limited training that the army mobilized them as Base Hospital No. 27 and shipped them off for further training under direct military supervision.[33] The Jefferson Medical College organized its volunteers and presented themselves as a body to the army, who designated them as Base Hospital No. 38.[34] The men from Pitt and Jefferson joined hundreds of others from across the state and the nation at Camp Crane in Allentown, Pennsylvania. Camp Crane was established in August 1917 as the home of the United States Army Ambulance Corps (USAAC, pronounced "you sack"). Other camps trained medical personnel, too, but only in addition to other training programs, for instance infantry training, while Camp Crane was the only base dedicated to training medical personnel. Camp Crane conditioned every category of men

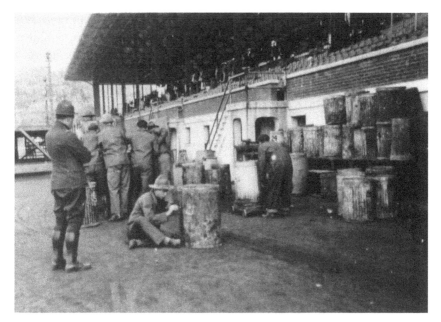

Soldiers at Camp Crane learning proper sanitary procedures, 1917. Camp Crane, Allentown, was the only military camp to train solely medical personnel during World War I. The U.S. Army Ambulance Corps, as well as physicians, were trained to army requirements. The camp also provided critical service to the state in October–November 1918 during the influenza epidemic. (Courtesy of the Lehigh County Historical Society.)

in the medical corps, from well-educated physicians who hailed from major centers of medical research and practice across the country, to stretcher bearers. By war's end, more than twenty thousand soldiers either trained at Camp Crane or billeted temporarily on their way to troop ships in New York.[35]

Wartime demands stretched Pennsylvania's medical infrastructure beyond its breaking point. The stress might be glimpsed by noting that roughly 33 percent of nurses and 25 percent of physicians had joined the military by the fall of 1918.[36] In their stead, women throughout the commonwealth volunteered as nurses, with the Red Cross by far the largest of the nursing organizations.[37] Volunteers took a short course, generally a few weeks, in nursing basics. Though by no means as well trained as nurses from conventional schools, the volunteers did vital work as visiting nurses, private home nurses, and in hospitals. Women physicians were not allowed to join the regular military medical services, but they performed valuable service through a host of national and military reserve physicians' organizations. Several graduates of Philadelphia's Women's Medical College of Pennsylvania, for instance Rosalie Slaughter, were conspicuous in their efforts on behalf of their soldier-patients and the rights of their fellow medical women to serve the country alongside, and equal to, their male counterparts.[38]

The shortage of personnel was exacerbated by additional demands placed on local and state public health resources. B. Franklin Royer, for instance, was called on to devise and oversee mosquito control efforts around what would become the Hog Island shipbuilding facility. For months Royer directed the excavation of small canals, the clearing of old pumps and the siting of new ones to drain hundreds of acres of swamp, with Royer's final task the spraying of kerosene on any standing water near the future dry docks to smother mosquito larvae.[39] As Royer controlled one source of disease along the Delaware, Wilmer Krusen, Philadelphia's director of public health, felt increased pressure from the navy to control another source of disease: the thousands of prostitutes and dozens of brothels that operated near the waterfront. Krusen urged and gained the passage of city ordinances that forced prostitutes in police custody to undergo examinations for venereal disease and treatment, if necessary, and used the limited resources of his department, with additional help from the city police and the navy's shore patrol, to close, or at least temporarily restrain, brothels.[40]

Influenza

Rates of pneumonia and deaths from it spiraled upward across the state during the war years, 1915–1918.[41] Pneumonia found ready purchase in the underfed, overworked, and obscenely housed industrial workforce. Spread by droplets exhaled by infected people, pneumonia was exceedingly difficult to treat and ranked as the greatest killer in the early twentieth century. While increased rates of pneumonia morbidity and mortality in crowded conditions are expected, the situation is complicated for historians and epidemiologists to analyze because, at some time not precisely determined as of this writing, a novel influenza virus entered the human population. The virus, according to the latest research, jumped from a bird to a mammal, perhaps a pig, and then entered the human population. The virus spent its time in its first mammalian host adapting to mammals' bodies. The virus then leapt, probably in China, to humans.[42]

For months, the infection the virus caused seemed to register on most nations' health statistics as a relatively highly infectious flu with lethality not markedly higher than normal flu. Samples of the virus recovered from tissue samples of lethal cases of influenza during the first seven months of 1918 and examined during the twenty-first century underscore an important and chilling fact; victims who died in early 1918 were killed by a much more avian-like virus than victims who died in July, by which time the virus was essentially a fully human influenza virus.[43] The virus, under immune pressure in humans, adapted to the human body in just a few months, a feat of evolution that few organisms, save the influenza virus, can achieve.

The centrality of Pennsylvania to the story of the pandemic of influenza is such that scarcely a history written about the catastrophe fails to mention the state and several of its cities and mining regions as important examples of the virus's ferociousness. Indeed, Philadelphia may have been the first place in which a virulent strain of the virus that was also highly infectious was documented by physicians. On June 22, 1918, a small British passenger ship, *City of Exeter*, pressed into service as a merchantman during the war, dropped anchor at the quarantine station on the Delaware River below Philadelphia.[44] The vessel departed England from Liverpool June 9, made no stops, and had no contact with other vessels.[45] Five days after leaving port, the first sailor reported ill, followed in rapid succession by dozens of others. The sickness produced fever and severe body aches, a dry cough, and for twenty-five men, a galloping pneumonia. Philadelphia's director of health, Krusen, in concert with the British consul, took the sickest men off the vessel and directly to Pennsylvania Hospital, where a group of eminent physicians from the University of Pennsylvania treated them. If H1N1 influenza virus, the agent of the later pandemic, had caused the sickness on *City of Exeter*, it failed to spread to the medical personnel who cared for them. In July and early August more ships carrying very ill sailors arrived in New York.

August proved to be the fatal month in the growing pandemic. In that month, virulent, highly infectious influenza established itself in Africa, Europe, and North America over the course of just two weeks. North America's first major, sustained outbreak occurred at the end of August in Boston. Philadelphia had its first cases in the Navy Yard by September 2.[46] The disease smoldered in the city for three weeks until September 28, when the city's enormous Fourth Liberty Loan Parade exponentially accelerated the spread of the virus. By October 5, more than eleven hundred lay dead in the city.[47] The virus emerged in Pittsburgh by mid-September, though its spread was far less spectacular than in Philadelphia. The virus infected progressively smaller communities, with most cities larger than twenty-five thousand infected by October 1. The smallest villages were all infected by mid-October, and villages close to a city a good deal earlier. In just two weeks the entire state plunged into illness at precisely the moment its medical resources reached their ebb.

The American medical infrastructure was really a patchwork of regulations and quality that varied tremendously between the forty-eight states. The federal government possessed little power to promulgate or enforce medical or sanitary standards, while nothing that remotely resembled the virus-hunting capabilities of the Centers for Disease Control existed. States and municipalities that invested few resources in public health programs or lacked hospitals and physicians stood to suffer most. So, too, did communities whose economies depended on steel mills and coal mines, as such work exposed laborers and their families to dangerous particulates that damaged lungs and bronchial passages and left sufferers vulnerable to the full array of respiratory disease.

Pennsylvania, unfortunately, had both of those shortcomings. On the one hand, the state department of health made great strides to ameliorate health threats in the rural areas and small towns. Yet many such communities did not have homegrown organizations charged with responding to an outbreak and relied instead on the state department of health. The arrangement worked well enough until 1918, but it had not been tested in the face of a truly state-wide epidemic; the last epidemic, cholera, had occurred in the 1830s and 1840s. The state department was not designed—indeed no state health body was ever designed—to respond simultaneously in every community that lacked a board of health. Furthermore, Pennsylvania's economy depended on just the sort of industry that was most damaging to respiratory systems—namely, iron and steel mills and mining. The textile industry, too, compromised the health of respiratory systems. The mills and mines not only harmed the health of workers directly engaged in those trades but also undermined the health of entire communities as the smoke and dust that poured from the furnaces and coke ovens blanketed towns and cities. Miners and breaker boys, meanwhile, brought home mineral dust to their families by way of their work clothes. In either case, particulate pollution infiltrated the bodies of people not employed by industrial works. Today, scientists call the respiratory problems recorded in such groups co-morbidities; they exist in a community before a disease like influenza appears, and they aid diseases like influenza in their deadly work.

In the wake of the death of Samuel Dixon in February 1918, the governor named B. Franklin Royer acting commissioner of health. As the epidemic built in Pennsylvania throughout September, Royer surveyed possible responses to the growing threat. On October 4, the acting commissioner settled on a course of action and announced the most comprehensive and stringent suite of state-level countermeasures against the epidemic in the nation. Royer's order banned all crowds associated with amusements, including any establishment that sold alcohol, athletic contests, and theaters and dance halls of any kind. The authority for Royer to issue such a sweeping order, which shuttered huge swaths of the state's economy, was found in the legislation that brought the department of health into being more than a decade earlier. Royer allowed local health boards and municipal governments to decide whether other measures, most importantly the closing of schools and places of worship, were in order.

In addition to the ban on crowds, Royer tirelessly coordinated flying squads of nurses and medical students, as well as a small number of physicians, and sent them to the worst-hit rural areas, many of which lacked physicians during even nonepidemic years. Perhaps his most incredible feat was gaining the cooperation of military authorities for the release of men from Camp Crane to assist in the small towns and rural districts of eastern Pennsylvania. The aid the camp sent was substantial: 851 enlisted men, including ambulance drivers and crews who used their army-issued ambulances to carry them to stricken coal towns, as well as orderlies and stretcher-bearers.[48] Camp Crane also sent 125 physicians, easily the largest group of physicians to come under Royer's direction during the epidemic.

The horror in the coal communities was captured by writer John O'Hara, who was born in the coal region town of Pottsville and was one of the exceedingly few authors to utilize the epidemic as a vehicle for their writing. O'Hara, a teenager during the epidemic, assisted his physician father in his duties and commented that "young men who already wheezed with miner's asthma in their twenties stood no chance against the flu when it came to their little coal patch."[49] Entire families lay ill with no prospect of medical care in shanty towns on the edges of the coal fields. While thousands of miners and their family members died in their hovels, many of those who survived owed their lives to members of the U.S. Army Ambulance Corps—the USAACs—and to Royer and the department of health that organized and oversaw their efforts.

The noble efforts of the state department of health notwithstanding, the battle against influenza was mostly a local affair carried on by municipal public health authorities with resources already present in a community, for instance donated tents and blankets, and whatever drugs, aspirin for instance, that were in stock at pharmacies. In the context of local responses, women, whether trained or volunteer nurses, shouldered the majority of the burden of treating the ill and comforting the dying. In Philadelphia roughly three thousand nuns volunteered for nursing duty. They served the community in emergency and regular hospitals, while they formed the backbone of the city's effort to send nurses into neighborhoods to visit homes filled with the sick and supervise their care.[50] Statewide, roughly three hundred emergency hospitals opened, with nine hundred doctors assigned to service in them.[51] However, with medical care in the case of influenza limited to palliative treatment, the majority of the work in the emergency hospitals was accomplished by nine hundred registered nurses and three thousand volunteers, the vast majority of them women.

Nowhere was the overwhelming power of the epidemic better exemplified than in Pennsylvania's largest city. The course of the epidemic in Philadelphia has become infamous in the annals of the pandemic for the speed with which the virus smothered the city and overwhelmed its resources. By October 7, authorities estimated that roughly two hundred thousand people were ill with influenza or pneumonia and more fell ill with each passing minute. Hospitals throughout the city found themselves overwhelmed and placed patients in hallways and offices. The city department of health established ten emergency hospitals but found very few people with enough training or courage to staff them. Another problem, that of corpses laying for days in homes and apartments, to say nothing of a city morgue stacked with five hundred putrefying bodies, taxed the city further, while the smell of decay drained the morale of citizens.

Frustrated and with no alternatives, Krusen asked the Roman Catholic Archdiocese of Philadelphia on October 8 to assume responsibility for epidemic control in the city.[52] Within days the diocese sent hundreds of nuns to run the emergency hospitals and act as visiting nurses, especially in the homes of the poor, regardless of religion, color, or ethnicity. Priests and seminary students removed hundreds of bodies from homes and hundreds more from the city morgue and buried them, often in trench graves that snaked across cemeteries such as Holy Cross and New Cathedral cemeteries. Though the dying continued apace, and actually grew worse during the week that followed the church's response, the terror diminished with the removal and burial of bodies and the rational management of the emergency hospitals. By the end of November a staggering number of people, at least fifteen thousand, were dead. No major city in America suffered a breakdown as complete as Philadelphia's.

Pittsburgh suffered an even higher mortality rate from influenza/pneumonia during the epidemic than Philadelphia. Unlike Philadelphia, however, Pittsburgh's epidemic period lasted six months, easily the longest in the nation, and did not strain the city in the way that Philadelphia's outbreak, accelerated by its ill-timed parade, did. Instead, Pittsburgh, with the pulmonary health of its citizens already compromised by its sooty air, languished for months. The city's department of health, headed by William H. Davis, an accountant with no medical experience, and the mayor, who resented the intrusion of state officials and their mandatory crowd ban, spent much of the epidemic fighting against Royer and his proclamation. Surprisingly, a week after the crowd ban was enacted by the state and with hundreds of sick throughout the city, Davis informed reporters that "what constitutes an epidemic is a matter of opinion."[53] Pittsburgh, the quintessentially laissez-faire industrial metropolis, failed to close schools until weeks into the outbreak, opened only a few small emergency hospitals with fewer than four hundred beds for a city of six hundred thousand, and spent weeks fighting with the state commissioner of health for the right to end the crowd ban and resume alcohol sales. Though the state threatened to jail any saloon or theater owner who opened before the state ended the ban, the damage was already done. The virus, and the pneumonia-causing bacteria that gained purchase in lungs damaged by the virus and Pittsburgh soot, claimed thousands of victims through April 1919. The final toll probably exceeded six thousand deaths by May 1919, when the epidemic sputtered out. In all, Pennsylvania recorded more than 67,000 deaths between September 1 and December 31, 1918, making it not only the worst-hit state in the nation but the state with the three highest death rates nationally for large cities: Pittsburgh, Scranton, and Philadelphia, respectively.[54]

The end of the influenza epidemic also marked the end of the state department of health as a leading light in public health in the nation. Acting commissioner Royer, whose apolitical style of management irked the governor and other important Republicans, was replaced by Dr. Edward Martin. Martin earned his medical degree in 1883, just as the germ theory of disease debuted. His tenure, and of those who followed him through World War II, was characterized by a focus on preventive medicine, with especial care paid to medical examination of schoolchildren, continued control of tuberculosis, and inspection of restaurants, dairies, and other entities whose normal course of operations might affect the public's health. The control of narcotics, which might strike many twenty-first-century readers as a law enforcement function, actually fell primarily under the purview of the department of health, as well as local health boards.

Medicine, whether practiced by private doctors or hospitals, also entered a period of incremental growth in major discoveries and treatment options. For instance, the popularity of radiation as a cancer treatment increased, and new and more complicated surgeries were performed, but new antitoxins and vaccines did not emerge in the 1920s and 1930s. The most important new treatments were the various sulfonamides, or sulfa drugs. Sulfonamides were the first antibiotics and could be used to inhibit the infection of wounds as well as against bacterial infections within the body. Though not as effective against a wide class of bacteria as penicillin and other antibiotics, they were an important step in reducing deaths and time of convalescence from many bacterial infections and saved many lives in Pennsylvania through the end of World War II.

Conclusion

Pennsylvania medicine rapidly came of age during the early twentieth century. In every category—medical education, entry of women and African Americans into the medical professions, research, and public health—the state improved. What is more, though its medical schools and hospitals faced increased competition for students and physicians from a wave of university and hospital openings in other states at the turn of the twentieth century, Pennsylvania actually increased its capacity to educate physicians and nurses and offer the best possible care throughout the period. Yet with all of the advances in medicine and increase in hospital space, as well as the advent of a rejuvenated state public health organization, the state failed miserably in its fight against the deadliest epidemic it ever faced. The death rates in the state's major cities, as well as its mining districts, were appalling and were to some degree, even with the drain of medical personnel by the war effort, unnecessary.

During the interwar period, Pennsylvania made incremental changes to its medical delivery system even as the role of public health transitioned from a rapid reaction force to combat epidemics, to enforcers of sanitary standards, standards that became increasingly easy to maintain as technology reduced the dangers associated with, for instance, contaminated water supplies. The next era of Pennsylvania's medical history emerged amid a climate of triumphant excitement surrounding the so-called end of infectious disease even as chronic illness carried an ever-increasing share of citizens to their deaths and new microbial threats emerged.

5

PROMISE AND PERIL OF PRIVATE MEDICINE,
1946–2017

THE END OF WORLD WAR II marked the beginning of a period of incredible economic growth for the nation and prosperity for American families, especially white, working- and middle-class families. The thirty-five years that followed the war resounded with a medical triumphalism unparalleled since the turn of the century, which marked the end of a great period of discoveries and practical benefits that flowed from them. Foremost among the innovations was penicillin, a term that denotes in the public mind both the name for a particular drug as well as a symbol of the first generation of antibiotics, including streptomycin and tetracycline. Viruses, too, saw their power curtailed as new vaccines that protected against influenza, measles, mumps, and rubella, as well as vaccinations against common bacterial infections such as diphtheria, tetanus, and pertussis, relegated once-terrifying infectious diseases to history. Chronic diseases associated with age and lifestyle, including heart disease, cancer, and diabetes, began their inexorable rise in the mortality charts as mortality rates from infectious disease diminished.

As the power of infectious disease declined, so too did the power of state and local public health bodies. Consider that in 1915, Pennsylvania employed quarantines and isolation to combat the spread of infectious disease, still found itself in the midst of purifying the water supplies of millions of citizens, and was fighting to ensure the protection of the food supply. Thirty years later, chlorine had banished waterborne illness, state and federal laws largely protected the food supply, and serious infectious disease was mostly avoidable or curable. Public health in Pennsylvania faded from public view as private medicine demanded a growing share of the power and money invested in healthcare. The preeminence of private medicine in the lives of the working and middle classes left to public health the responsibilities of caring for the poor and maintaining sanitary standards most people had long since come to accept as the norm. Private medicine dominated Pennsylvania's post–World War II healthcare system—aided by billions of dollars of tax money in the form of Medicare, Medicaid, and state grants to universities and research institutions, hospitals, and other programs. By the late twentieth century, a growing number of powerful, regional healthcare networks challenged the dominance of stand-alone hospitals in Pennsylvania's small cities and large towns, while alternative medicine, health clubs, the anti-vaccination movement, and the internet challenged the hegemony of conventional medicine in ways not seen since the mid-nineteenth century.

The benefits of better healthcare for Pennsylvanians belied the dangers that emerged throughout the period. Antibiotics, for instance, provoked bacteria to evolve defenses against humanity's new weapons. Other threats were recognized when pathogens hitherto unsuspected as the cause of disease unmasked their lethal potential, as in the case of the legionella and borrelia (Lyme disease) bacteria, or changed, as in the various epidemic iterations of influenza. The worst of the new threats, HIV, emerged in Pennsylvania in the late 1970s, long before doctors reported the first confirmed cases. By the turn of the twenty-first century, new challenges related to the growing elderly population in the state, as well as prescription opioid abuse, to say nothing of nicotine use, demanded a new fusion of public health and private medicine.

Antibiotic Revolution

The influenza pandemic that raged at the end of World War I prompted a wave of research on a disease discounted as a major cause of mortality. Much of the research revolved around the role of Pfeiffer's bacillus. Ever since German scientist Robert Pfeiffer had repeatedly isolated it in the nasal and throat secretions of influenza sufferers during the 1890s, it had been considered responsible for influenza. During the 1918–1919 pandemic, researchers had again isolated it in the secretions of influenza patients, but not in all or even in most patients. As this anomaly appeared to violate every principle of bacteriology, some scientists suspected that Pfeiffer's bacillus was not the causative agent of influenza but instead an opportunistic bacterium that used the damage caused by the true agent of influenza to thrive in the human respiratory tract. In the 1920s, Alexander Fleming, a scientist at St. Mary's Hospital, University of London, engaged himself in the growth and study of Pfeiffer's bacillus. The germ was notoriously difficult for even the most adept research-ers to culture and so, the story goes, Fleming arrived in his laboratory in September 1928 to find his petri dishes tainted with a common mold, *Peni-cillium notatum*. Fleming noticed that the cultures of bacteria he cultivated seemed constrained by *Penicillium*, though why was unclear. A poor writer and lecturer, Fleming was unable to convince the scientific community that his discovery ranked as one of the most important in the history of medicine, though a few researchers in the 1930s managed to cure test subjects of gon-orrhea and some streptococcus and staphylococcus infections using the chemical secreted by the mold. By the early 1940s, the efficacy of penicillin, as Fleming termed the chemical isolated from the mold, was understood and it began to be mass-produced as part of the war effort.

Penicillin moved quickly into the civilian market after the war and was joined by penicillin derivatives as well as streptomycin, an antibiotic derived from a bacterium found in soil. The effect of the new drugs was immediate and, to all appearances, constituted a finale to bacteria's reign of terror. This was especially the case with wound infections and the fatal gangrene and septicemia they so often caused. The standard procedure in such cases had been to apply salts and tubes to dry and drain the wound, sulfonamides to kill the bacteria, and excision of dead flesh and amputation of limbs in severe cases, which were numerous. Penicillin changed the landscape of wound treatment, as well as the treatment of pneumonia, a perennial killer of young and old alike. Streptomycin, released in the late 1940s, was capable of killing the bacterium that caused tuberculosis.

The changes brought to Pennsylvania medicine and public health by an-tibiotics were swift. Throughout the state hundreds of hospital beds normally occupied by patients sick with bacterial infections lay empty, and morbidity and mortality rates from postoperative infections plummeted. In Pittsburgh, the Municipal Hospital, attached to the University of Pittsburgh and mostly reserved for the care of infectious disease cases, stood nearly vacant by the late 1940s as even life-threatening infections required only a short hospital stay or were treated on an outpatient basis.[1] The same was true at Philadelphia's Municipal Hospital for Contagious Disease, which by the mid-1950s was renamed and remade into the Philadelphia General Hospital Northern Divi-sion to reflect its transformation from an isolation and treatment center to a general municipal hospital.

One of the most stunning antibiotic victories brought to a swift close a half century of state-run tuberculosis hospitals and dispensaries. Tuberculo-sis, one of the commonwealth's most feared infectious diseases through World War II, killed hundreds of thousands of Pennsylvanians over the course of two centuries. By the second decade of the twentieth century no other disease commanded as much of the state's resources, including typhoid, which was largely left to local authorities to eliminate. The state's chain of three large tuberculosis hospitals and dozens of clinics, run by a combined staff of thousands, constituted a sort of health department within the state's department of health. With the introduction of streptomycin in the late 1940s, however, the fight against tuberculosis drew to a quick, and seemingly final, close. Rather than long stretches of confinement in state sanatoria, indigent patients and those with advanced tuberculosis required a few months of antibiotics. Early cases of tuberculosis required even less intensive antibiotic therapy. Because of antibiotics, the chief goal of the state department of health transitioned from long-term care until recovery or death, to monitoring patients to ensure their compliance with the drug regimen. B. Franklin Royer, who began his career in public health managing a large isolation hospital, spent his final years adapting the state's tuberculosis control methods to the antibiotic era. In contrast to the thousands of patients institutionalized in the previous era, only those pulmonary tuberculosis sufferers who refused to follow the state's antibiotic protocol were forcibly isolated or jailed under Royer's revised methods.[2] The last state tuberculosis patients, mostly those who had spent years under the state's care and often suffered debilitating reduction of their lung capacity, were moved to private care facilities by the 1960s.

The power of antibiotics was augmented by the prophylactic power of municipal water treatment. Drinking water quality improved to thoroughly modern standards by 1946, by which time Pennsylvania's municipalities had constructed "1,500 chlorination plants and 457 sewage treatment plants."[3] The modern plants filtered the water and used chemicals to improve clarity and taste, but the most important ingredient in the process was chlorine, which destroyed the bacteria responsible for the full spectrum of gastrointestinal illness. Cleaning the state's water supplies resulted in a drop in typhoid mortality from about four thousand reported deaths in 1900 to just one death in 1960, and in the same period, deaths from four major categories of infectious waterborne illnesses declined from five thousand deaths to a mere thirteen.[4]

The extension of modern water treatment to even the smallest municipalities combined with antibiotics radically altered the public health landscape in America. The role of state and local public health authorities in Pennsylvania shifted from aggressive campaigns against infectious disease to the maintenance and updating of existing standards of sanitation and increased concentration on chronic illnesses. As a result, physicians engaged in public health work were increasingly viewed, especially after World War II, as lazy, or somehow inadequate. Pennsylvania's department of health might fairly be said to have begun transitioning away from an innovative, powerful disease-fighting institution earlier than the health departments of most states; the only head of the Pennsylvania's state department of health to have any preventive health experience after Samuel Dixon's death was B. Franklin Royer, who remained as acting commissioner of health for only a year.[5]

One threat that remained, however, and one which the state department of health had been charged with fighting, was environmental pollution. The department's charter made cleaning up the state's streams one of its chief, enumerated responsibilities. As the department discovered, however, reducing any sort of pollution in Pennsylvania pitted it against industrial interests whose profit was often based on their right to conduct their operations, including disposal of waste, in the cheapest possible manner. Pollution fouled huge swaths of the commonwealth's land, most of its surface waters, and burdened the air with soot. Millions of the state's residents lived and worked in an environment so degraded that today's Pennsylvanians can scarcely imagine the grim environment of the commonwealth's steel cities and coal towns.

Nowhere was the effect of pollution more evident to a great number of people than in Pittsburgh and the surrounding region. Pittsburgh's air had long alarmed public health authorities and reformers, some of whom took photographs of the city's downtown in broad daylight to highlight automobiles with headlights on to cut through ground level smog and the sides of buildings hidden from sight above just a few stories by thick tendrils of soot that wrapped around the city, invaded the lungs and the smallest capillaries, and damaged cells and the cardiopulmonary system.[6] Yet attempts by the state department of health to reduce air pollution, often termed smoke abatement, ran afoul of industry, legislators, and courts, and all efforts to reduce smoke languished until after the war, at which point the city's association with soot and grime had begun to affect its economic potential.

The mayoral election of 1946 brought David L. Lawrence and a plan for Pittsburgh that included drastic reduction in smoke from industrial operations. His Pittsburgh Renaissance urban plan married environmental reformers, before such a term existed, with big business and political leaders. Though most people are used to viewing industry and environmentalists on opposite sides, some prominent business leaders recognized that prospective executives fresh out of college were passing on positions with Pittsburgh firms simply because the city did not beckon as a place to raise families; it was said that young wives told their husbands that the sootiness of the city was repellent.

A 1948 disaster with both human and natural origins added urgency to smoke abatement in Pittsburgh. Over the course of five days in October, a temperature inversion over the town of Donora along the Monongahela River south of Pittsburgh trapped pollutants from a zinc smelting plant under a layer of warm air. Not only was the smog so dense that daylight driving was nearly impossible, but the soot contained high amounts of poisonous gases such as fluorine and sulfuric acid. Only rain abated the smog, and by then, twenty lay dead, half the population of the town of fourteen thousand reported respiratory distress, and within months, several dozen more died.[7] Even a decade later, death rates in Donora far exceeded the region's other industrial towns. The disaster led to the passage, in 1959, of a state law designed to empower state and local agencies to reduce and prohibit many forms of air pollution.

In addition to changes in the operations and goals of the state department of health, local health bodies, too, evolved. The township health officer virtually disappeared, replaced by the county health department, empowered to manage and respond to sanitary threats and outbreaks. The changes meant county departments often assumed responsibility for things like restaurant inspection, inspection of housing, and water safety, while the threat of outbreaks, especially ones with lethal consequences, shrank. The state and county both shifted their gaze to the health and safety of school children, with dental care, physical examinations, and early intervention a focus. Importantly, diagnosis of an ailment—be it poor eyesight, caries, or something more serious, like tuberculosis—often resulted in the parents seeking care from a private physician.

Along with the success of antibiotics against bacterial diseases, victories were won against a number of viral illnesses through the use of vaccines. No success was more important in terms of global and national health, or more intrinsically linked to Pennsylvania, than the polio vaccine. Polio outbreaks increased in the United States throughout the late nineteenth century and the first half of the twentieth century, due in large part to the cleaning of America's water supplies, which resulted in lower rates of exposure to the virus in the early months of life and growing susceptibility to the virus among people from birth through their teen years. The worst of the early epidemics, in 1916, presaged the nationwide epidemics of the 1940s and early 1950s. Not only could the virus paralyze legs as in the case of President Franklin Delano Roosevelt; it also had the power to paralyze the muscles responsible for respiration. The first breakthrough for such sufferers arrived in 1928 when Philip Drinker, who was born and spent much of his early life in Pennsylvania, first used his invention, the so-called iron lung, to save the life of a polio-stricken girl.[8] Though the iron lung saved thousands of lives, and some people used versions of the iron lung for decades to maintain their lives, mechanical devices were not a substitute for cures or prevention. When scientists determined that polio's cause was viral, a vaccine seemed the only possible prevention.

The quest for a polio vaccine accelerated immediately following World War II. The National Foundation for Infantile Paralysis (NFIP), better known as the March of Dimes, spearheaded the effort with money and by coordinating the research efforts of several teams. Jonas Salk at the University of Pittsburgh led one of the teams, and Albert Sabin at the University of Cincinnati led the Pittsburgh team's chief rival. Salk came to the University of Pittsburgh in 1947 from the University of Michigan at a time when the city and the university were relative medical backwaters. Salk later admitted that, were it not for the fact that he "fell in love" with the grimy city, its "provincialism," as Salk termed it, would have prevented him from accepting the position.[9] To his affection for Pittsburgh one might add that the opportunity to inaugurate and direct a new virology program at only thirty-two years of age must also have been a strong pull. Private sources of funding were few in the city as Pittsburgh's wealthy families tended to spend their charity either in the city on projects unrelated to higher education or in fashionable cities like New York and Chicago. Fortunately, both private donors and the NFIP allowed Salk to expand his facilities, purchase new equipment, and add scientists and assistants.

The NFIP's first move in its systematic effort to develop a vaccine was to type, or identify, the different strains of polio virus. Gathering as much information as possible about the viruses allowed Salk and the others to identify the most virulent strains and clarified the degree of cross immunity that infection with one strain offered against other polio viruses. Salk proved particularly adept at isolating strains because much of his prior work at both the University of Michigan and in the army during World War II included identifying different strains of the influenza virus in humans and animals. After the major strains of polio were identified, the next step was to develop a safe vaccine. Two possibilities existed: a vaccine that relied on killed virus or one produced from a weakened but living virus. Salk favored a killed virus vaccine because earlier tests with vaccines and solutions produced with live virus caused severe illness, paralysis, and even death among test subjects, including children.

The meticulous, single-minded drive of Salk to create a polio vaccine is legendary. After his exhaustive typing of polio strains, he moved to attenuating polio virus in baths of chemicals, including formaldehyde, to completely inactivate—kill—viruses. The inactive viruses still aroused an immune response, which allowed the body to produce immune memory cells that responded to the signature of the viruses and that would readily identify and eliminate the virus when it entered the body through subsequent natural infection. By late 1954 Salk believed he had perfected a safe vaccine and began clinical trials on tens of thousands of people, mostly children. Salk revealed later that his own wife and children received doses of the experimental vaccine.

On April 9, 1955, a national public proclamation announced that a safe, effective vaccine for polio had been developed by the University of Pittsburgh and its brilliant but obscure head of virology, Jonas Salk. In one fell swoop, Salk was a household name across the country and around the world while the University of Pittsburgh basked in its new prestige as a center of medical research. Salk remains the single most famous medical researcher produced by Pennsylvania. In the wake of his discovery, and the realization that countless millions of children no longer faced paralysis and death from polio, the state legislature struck a medal to commemorate Salk and awarded him an endowed professorship at the university. Salk, who eschewed the limelight whenever possible, went as far as to refuse to patent the vaccine because he believed any barrier to the swiftest possible distribution of the vaccine an unthinkable offense against humanity.[10]

The Microbes Strike Back

The mid-1960s marked important transitions in Pennsylvania health and medicine. The Great Society program of President Lyndon B. Johnson included Medicare and Medicaid. The former covered much of the medical costs for senior citizens, while Medicaid covered the costs of healthcare for the poor. The programs did not force people to use public health doctors; rather, private physicians and hospitals treated patients, many of them heretofore too poor to afford the services of a physician. A few years after the passage of Johnson's programs, President Richard M. Nixon declared war on cancer. All of these programs and declarations signaled that America, and Pennsylvania, was in the middle of an important health transition wherein deaths from infectious disease fell to the bottom of the mortality rankings while chronic diseases such as cancer and heart disease claimed the largest share of deaths, usually in people of advanced age. Yet even nations that cleaned their water supplies and seemed to have eradicated childhood diseases faced new microbial threats that began to emerge from around the world.

Though these microbial threats were far removed from Pennsylvania, it was foolish to believe that pathogens would be chained so easily by human ingenuity or that Pennsylvania could remain untouched. One weapon the microbes possessed was the oldest tool all organisms use to thwart threats to their existence—evolution. The moment humans initiated the use of antibiotics, bacteria began to evolve defenses against them. Bacteria that survived a course of antibiotics tended to be precisely the bacteria whose progeny would be most likely to survive even higher doses of antibiotics in the future. Changes occurred in bacterial cell walls, cellular pumps to eject antibiotics developed, and in some cases bacteria even fed on antibiotics, all of which thwarted to some degree medicine's most effective measure against their survival. The dosage of antibiotics given for simple throat and ear infections, for instance, began to rise as early as the 1950s as one strain of bacteria after another gained strength against an increasing array of antibiotics. By the turn of the twenty-first century, antibiotic strains of tuberculosis appeared that effectively resisted every drug on the market and reduced physicians to providing palliative care, just as they had only sixty years earlier. Authorities began to openly worry that an age was approaching when many common bacteria would be susceptible to only a small handful of very powerful, very expensive antibiotics.

Evolutionary changes also enabled some families of viruses to pose a constant threat to Pennsylvanians. The most important of these viruses were the type A influenza viruses. Influenza A viruses are most responsible for the sickness and death attributed to both seasonal and epidemic influenza. Influenza viruses are inherently bad at making exact copies of themselves, and this mutability allows the viruses to rapidly evolve, with changes that allow it to hide from the human immune system. In 1956, for example, a novel influenza virus emerged in China and sparked the 1957–1958 Asian flu pandemic, while another influenza virus emerged in Hong Kong in 1968 and caused the Hong Kong influenza pandemic. Both outbreaks circled the globe and killed thousands of Pennsylvanians. However, antibiotics prevented opportunistic bacteria from establishing themselves in lungs and causing fatal, secondary bacterial pneumonia.[11]

Viruses are also capable of lurking in the background of the environment, usually in animals, and causing disease, even fatal disease, without arousing suspicion. Such viruses may cause sudden epidemics that force people to recognize a new threat to their health. Cases of viruses that moved from mere background levels of interference in human health to epidemic status happened often between the early 1950s and mid-1970s as people pushed deeper into undeveloped land and upset ecosystems that kept viral host animals, and the viruses they carried, in check. For instance, hantavirus emerged near the Hantaan River in South Korea among American troops in 1951, and Junin emerged in Argentina, Machupo in Bolivia, and Lassa in Africa.[12] All emerged in rural areas and all were spread by mice. In 1976, Ebola emerged in a rural Zaire village hospital, its viral reservoir still unknown in the early twenty-first century, though suspicion rests on several species of bat. During the same year, other microbes in and around Philadelphia suddenly appeared, killed dozens, and frightened the entire nation.

Especial importance was attached to the year 1976 for Pennsylvania and the nation, as it marked the bicentennial of the signing and adoption of the Declaration of Independence in Philadelphia. Though no one could have suspected it when the year began, 1976 also marked an important year in the history of Pennsylvania medicine. Two outbreaks that year, one near Philadelphia and the other within the city, undermined the complacency people had shown for three decades to infectious disease. The first outbreak began in February when a young soldier stationed at Fort Dix, New Jersey, only forty miles from Philadelphia and twenty miles from the border with Pennsylvania, collapsed and went into respiratory failure during a march. Transported to hospital, the young man died within days as a number of other soldiers on the base fell ill. Tests on the dead soldier and his sick comrades pointed to an influenza virus—namely, H1N1, often referred to as swine flu—as the culprit. Health authorities warned President Gerald Ford that the virus isolated in Fort Dix was related to the virus that caused the 1918–1919 pandemic.

In response, authorities won approval for a crash program of vaccine development and distribution. The virus ultimately failed to cause infections beyond the perimeter of the base, but tens of millions of people received the vaccine and attention was once again thrown on the dangers of influenza. In Philadelphia, newspapers printed stories that detailed the travails of the city during the 1918 epidemic. The papers also sought survivors of the outbreak in 1918 and published their recollections. One woman in her eighties related that her husband died in 1918 after only a few days' illness. Because she could not find someone to take the body for either embalming or burial, she placed the corpse in a corner of the home and placed a cloth over it. After a few days passed, men came to retrieve the body and upon removing the cloth, she found her husband's face crawling with flies and maggots.[13] Such recollections reinforced the seriousness of influenza in Dix and the threat it posed to Pennsylvania and the nation.

Through the summer of 1976, the swine flu scare increased even as Philadelphia basked in bicentennial celebrations. Among the groups that selected

Philadelphia as a conference location during that auspicious year was the Pennsylvania wing of the American Legion. Hundreds of Legionnaires flooded the Bellevue-Stratford Hotel for several days of Legion business and good times with old friends. Within a few days of its end, a dozen Legionnaires died in their homes or community hospitals, sometimes of apparent heart attacks. By a stroke of luck, two of the dozen earliest victims went to the same family doctor in Bloomsburg. When the doctor realized that both of these men attended the conference, he alerted the state department of health to the potential danger. The health department initiated an investigation, but unlike a half century earlier when the state would have entirely handled the growing outbreak, perhaps with aid from the city and university labs, it was the federal government, specifically the Centers for Disease Control and Prevention, that led the way.

With headlines across the state and throughout the nation blaring news of the mounting epidemic, an epidemic with possible, even probable, connections to swine flu, people began to suspect that perhaps the two dozen dead Legionnaires were the first victims of a coming influenza pandemic.[14] Curiously, though, by the end of August, without a pathogen identified, the epidemic burned out. It was not until December 1976 that the pathogen, *Legionella pneumophila*, was isolated by CDC scientists. State and federal epidemiologists then linked the bacteria to water inside the air conditioning cooling towers of the hotel. Legionnaires' disease continues to cause thousands of reported illnesses every year in the country, and as recently as 2011–2012 two dozen patients were sickened, and six died, in a Legionnaires' outbreak in a Pittsburgh Veterans Affairs hospital.[15]

Five years after the outbreaks of swine flu and Legionnaires' scared Pennsylvania and the nation, 1981 reports from Los Angeles in June and New York City in July indicated that young, otherwise healthy homosexual men were developing and dying from rare forms of pneumonia and skin cancer. The reports are recognized by scholars as the first alert of a new sickness. Within a year the CDC and others realized that a new pandemic was circling the globe. By the mid-1980s a new pathogen, human immunodeficiency virus (HIV), was identified as causing a new disease, acquired immunodeficiency syndrome (AIDS). The virus found its way from person to person through unsafe sexual practices, intravenous drug use, and blood transfusions. Pennsylvania offered ample opportunity for HIV to spread.

In a classic example of economic dislocation leading to deprivation, disease, and death, important parts of the state's economic underpinnings, including coal mining, the ferrous metals industry, and the large and small urban centers that depended on heavy industry, declined during the 1960s and 1970s. As prosperous families, usually white, moved to suburban communities, once-vibrant mill towns were emptied of their inhabitants. Pittsburgh and Philadelphia each lost hundreds of thousands of residents, and in both cities huge swaths of housing were left nearly uninhabited. The people who remained constituted some of the poorest in the state, forced to eke out a living through a combination of low-paying, low-skill jobs; government assistance; and crime, including prostitution and drug distribution.

By the late 1980s, an infectious disease was once again in the first rank of killers in Pennsylvania's two largest cities; this time it was AIDS. What many do not realize is that it also became one of the primary killers of people in the state's declining industrial towns. Across the state, as across the country, an entire generation of hemophiliacs, intravenous drug users, and prostitutes was wiped out. Homosexuals, especially young men, faced very high fatality rates, too. Responses in Pennsylvania to the AIDS crisis varied, but religious beliefs and attitudes toward homosexuals, drug users, and minorities all influenced public opinion and the response of state and local officials. Across the state, in a perfect example of nonscientific beliefs guiding public health policy, groups fought against needle exchange programs; the message of safe, or at least safer, sex through the use of condoms; and other public health responses to an untreatable, but rather easily preventable, disease. In the face of such opposition, much of it colored by overt homophobia and racism, groups dedicated to fighting the spread of AIDS were galvanized by the deaths of loved ones, including an increasing number of working- and middle-class heterosexuals stricken and killed by HIV. The groups demanded money for research on the virus and the development of treatments and, eventually, a vaccine.

All of the major research institutions and hospitals in the state participated in drug development and trials, and received millions of dollars from state and local taxpayers, as well as private donors and research foundations, for the urgent work. By the mid-1990s, researchers had hit on a combination of retroviral and immune-supporting drugs that cleared HIV from the bloodstream and reduced overall viral load (the amount of virus per unit of blood) to amounts not detectable by tests—amounts so low, in fact, that passing the virus on through sex and even the sharing of needles was deemed almost impossible. The retroviral therapy regime, announced publicly in 1996, did not offer a cure; to keep the virus at bay meant lifelong use of the drugs, some of which provoked debilitating and even fatal complications in patients. Two decades after its introduction, the drug therapy remained the best way to save life and limit spread of the virus. The search for a vaccine continues in the early twenty-first century. From the late 1970s to 2015, the virus had killed tens of thousands of Pennsylvanians.

Medical Leviathan

The healthcare industry evolved into arguably the single biggest piece of Pennsylvania's economy before the end of the twentieth century. The transformation of medicine from a loose network of community hospitals, private physicians, and a few mostly university-related research institutions into an economic behemoth responsible for more than $17 billion worth of economic activity in the state during 2014 alone is a decades-long tale of an ever-greater share of private and public resources devoted to preventing and caring for the sick, and finding ways to pay for care that became progressively more sophisticated and expensive.

Pennsylvania added several medical and osteopathic schools, including Hershey, which functioned as the medical school of Penn State University; the Drexel School of Medicine, in Philadelphia, which absorbed the Women's Medical College; and the Lake Erie College of Osteopathic Medicine, which ranks as one of the largest medical schools in the nation. Beyond the growth in the state's number of medical schools—only New York, California, and Texas are home to more than Pennsylvania—the quality of the state's medical schools increased uniformly, as did the quality of care offered by hospitals associated with medical schools. The excellence of the University of Pennsylvania's School of Medicine (since 2011 the Perelman School of Medicine) is exemplified by its consistent recognition as one of the top ten medical schools in the nation.[16] Of even greater importance are its network of hospitals, several of which rank as among the best in the world, including Children's Hospital of Philadelphia, regarded by many as the world's greatest children's hospital, and the Hospital of the University of Pennsylvania, generally recognized as one of the top twenty hospitals in the nation.[17]

Throughout the twentieth century, the University of Pittsburgh continued to enhance its facilities and faculty. The same kind of effort that brought Salk to the campus in 1947 continued to attract money and change the perception of the university, its medical school, and the hospitals connected to the university, though even in the early 1960s people of means usually traveled to Philadelphia or New York for medical care. The medical school's growth received an inestimable boost when Thomas Detre, a tenured professor in psychiatry at the Yale School of Medicine, agreed to head the Western Psychiatric Institute and Clinic and chair the school's psychiatry department.

By 1984 Detre was vice chancellor of the university and in a position to apply a model of self-funding that relied on moving profits derived from clinical practice, that is, proceeds from caring for patients, to fund research. The advances derived from research were then quickly moved into the clinical setting to enhance patient care and outcomes. Better quality of care attracted larger numbers of patients, who fed more money into research and ultimately received better care. By 2016–2017, the University of Pittsburgh School of Medicine ranked as one of the best medical schools in the nation and was a top ten recipient of research funding from the National Institutes of Health between 1997 and 2017.[18]

Closely aligned with the fortunes of the university's medical school was the progress at the University of Pittsburgh Medical Center, which functioned as the clinical arm of the university. The university, its medical school, and Presbyterian Hospital became loosely affiliated at the turn of the twentieth century. By the 1930s, the university began to act in partnership with a half dozen hospitals, all of which either relocated to or had a major presence in the Oakland section of the city where the university had been located since 1908. During the 1970s and 1980s, the influence of Detre and the power of the university meant the University of Pittsburgh, not the associated hospitals, dominated the administration, and the strategic vision, of the consortium. During the 1990s, UPMC, as it was officially titled in 1990, aggressively expanded its reach by buying community hospitals in the region and constructing its own health insurance, and then contracting with hospitals in its growing network to accept UPMC health insurance.

In 1998, to shield the university from financial liability, the University of Pittsburgh and UPMC separated from one another, though a series of formal agreements, informal practices, mutual obligations, and shared board members make the university responsible for teaching and research, while UPMC handles all aspects of patient treatment.[19] The expansion of UPMC, as the largest provider of medicine in western Pennsylvania, came at the price of competing hospitals and health systems, and resulted in antitrust lawsuits and legal wrangling between it and the city of Pittsburgh, which wanted a close examination of UPMC's tax-exempt status.

Regional healthcare networks also expanded rapidly at the turn of the twenty-first century. The logic for the expansion of regional centers is simple economics; stand-alone hospitals do not provide the flexibility that a network of hospitals provides. The Lehigh Valley, fifty miles northwest of Philadelphia with a population of about a half million by the year 2000, is one area that experienced the rise and domination of two health networks: St. Luke's University Health Network and Lehigh Valley Health Network. St. Luke's dominated healthcare in Bethlehem for decades, while the Lehigh Valley Health Network, which traces its beginnings to the opening of Allentown Hospital in 1898, held sway in Allentown. By the early 1970s, Lehigh Valley invested in a large, new suburban campus and within ten years was the largest provider of healthcare in the valley. During the early twentieth century, Lehigh Valley opened another large campus in Bethlehem, the traditional territory of St. Luke's Hospital. At roughly the same time, St. Luke's opened a campus in the heart of Allentown and both networks acquired smaller regional health networks and hospitals. By 2017, Lehigh Valley and St. Luke's were the number one and number two employers, respectively, in the Lehigh Valley.[20]

The Future

Pennsylvania's future as an international and national center of medical education and healthcare delivery is secure—for the time being. Pennsylvania, however, does face a number of challenges beyond the confines of health and medicine that will stress the commonwealth's health infrastructure in the near future. The state's population is aging, a fact that is coupled with a troubling trend in Pennsylvania's demography, namely the flight of a significant portion of the most educated and affluent eighteen- to forty-year-olds to other states. If the trend does not end, or if it speeds up, an increasing portion of Pennsylvania's population will face the health challenges of old age with a shrinking base of taxpayers to support their needs. An aging population also presents challenges with respect to seasonal influenza, as about 95 percent of annual influenza-related deaths are in those aged sixty-five years and older. Uncertainty surrounding Medicaid, Medicare, and the Affordable Care Act, to say nothing of prescription coverage for seniors and the poor, contribute to making the healthcare market increasingly more expensive relative to inflation and wages.[21]

The growth of regional and even state-spanning health networks is likely to continue for the foreseeable future. The efficiencies inherent in health networks when compared to single hospitals are too obvious to ignore. When a network also constructs health insurance, a health maintenance organization (HMO), or both to complement its services, the combination is often irresistible. At the same time, private practice physicians in some communities have found it all but impossible to function without at least some ties to local health networks. The corporate framework of the networks adds to concerns voiced by patients that their doctors spend little time with them, with a consequent erosion of the doctor-patient relationship. A personal relationship between physician and patient is not scientifically required to deliver

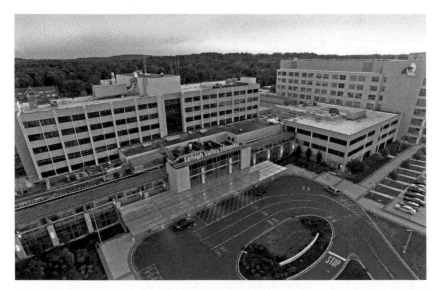

The Cedar Crest campus of Lehigh Valley Health Network, 2016. This campus is a direct outgrowth of the founding of Allentown Hospital in 1899. LVHN is now a large regional medical center with wings for cancer treatment, a trauma center with integrated helicopter transport, a burn unit, and medical research capacity. (Courtesy of Lehigh Valley Health Network.)

medicine, but it is needed to build the genuine trust and understanding that humanizes the delivery of care and results in a medicine far superior to the "assembly line" sort of medicine many patients have come to detest.[22] Patient backlash against what is perceived as impersonal care mirrors the sentiments people expressed a century and a half earlier, when allopathic medicine undermined the hold the many irregular schools of medicine enjoyed. The modern popularity of homeopathy, herbal, Ayurvedic, and other forms of unconventional and non-Western medical practices in part reflects the continued mistrust some feel for modern medicine.

The state's public health infrastructure faces a number of pressing concerns. In the short to medium term, terrorism and the inability to predict if, and exactly how, a terrorist strike might unfold in Pennsylvania, whether by a release of chemicals or bioweapons, or a nuclear or conventional bomb, makes constructing responses difficult. Opioid deaths, whether by heroin or prescription drugs, killed record numbers of Pennsylvanians in 2016 and 2017. Though opioid addiction presents a threat to the public health, the crisis demands a new approach to pain management among the state's physicians. A new sort of partnership between public health officials, physicians, and law enforcement is a necessary step to reducing access to narcotics and a reduction in addiction and deaths. The inevitable sudden outbreaks of infectious disease demand that the state's public health resources and its health networks, hospitals, and medical personnel remain capable of responding in both the near and long term. The epidemic threats of Legionnaires' and swine flu in the 1970s, replaced by AIDS in the 1980s, were themselves largely replaced in the public's mind by anthrax in 2001, another round of swine flu that killed hundreds of the state's citizens in 2009 and 2010, and the specter of Ebola disembarking at the Philadelphia or Pittsburgh airports in 2014–2015. Through all of its coming challenges, Pennsylvania must continue to augment its health resources while it educates its most important asset—its citizens—for a better, healthier future.

CONCLUSION

Keeping the Commonwealth Healthy

T HE GRAND SWEEP of Pennsylvania's medical past encompassed almost every major development in medicine, outbreak of disease, and public health. Yet the commonwealth's history of medicine is a unique story that reflects Pennsylvania's singular colonial roots, its development as an industrial power, the building of its medical and public health infrastructure, the incredible cultural diversity of its population, and the nature and course of the threats to the state's health.

The colonial beginnings of Pennsylvania medicine encompassed a period whose theories of disease and medicine were little changed from those espoused by people who lived in medieval London or ancient Rome. As primitive as our ancestors' notions may appear to the twenty-first-century observer, the great medical center of colonial Philadelphia had already by the mid-eighteenth century begun to offer glimpses of the trajectory the city and its people would chart during the next hundred years; a public health apparatus grew more complex, centers of medical education and debate flourished, and healthcare workers of every stripe confronted a long list of environmental and microbial threats. The rest of Pennsylvania, too, trod a path that it would follow for decades—one that saw its communities dependent on physicians with little training and no hospitals.

Perhaps the most fascinating part about the history of medicine in the state is its local nature. There is no need to visit a particular battlefield or mill as one would to learn the martial or industrial history of the state. Instead, disease and medicine fought one another in every home, imbued an entire subculture of the Pennsylvania Dutch with a sense of secret knowledge and an affirmation of their closely held religious beliefs, inspired innovation and hope, and caused grief. A walk through a pre-1920 cemetery, if one pays attention to the years that occur most frequently on the memorial stones, offers a glimpse into the life-and-death struggle our ancestors waged when confronted with epidemics. The contours of a community's history are written on the tombstones; 1793, 1832, and 1918 are years mostly forgotten by the present but representative of struggles as momentous, and usually far more lethal, than the death experienced on Pennsylvania's battlefields or during labor disputes.

The history of medicine continues to grow in the sense that more scholars recognize the importance of disease and medicine in the general narrative of the past. The next step is for the public to understand the vital importance of defining many of the most important events of Pennsylvania's history. The subtle impact of disease often confounds the casual observer of the state's past: What might have been had Native Americans not been decimated by disease? What effect did disease have on the Revolutionary War considering that disease at Valley Forge killed far more Continental soldiers than the battles of Germantown and Brandywine combined, and that Washington's troops were far better off than their British counterparts in the face of smallpox because of his orders to inoculate new soldiers? How did the lives of Pennsylvanians change in the wake of the most overlooked loss of life in the state's history—the influenza epidemic of 1918–1919? How has AIDS changed our discussions and views of sex, love, politics, and marriage? How will the state, its families and its government, cope with a rapidly graying population? The history of medicine in our state, then, is not a static event bordered by our memories; rather, medicine and disease inform our present, and its implications stretch into the far distant future.

AFTERWORD

COVID-19 in Pennsylvania

AS *THE HEALTH OF THE COMMONWEALTH* GOES TO PRESS, Pennsylvania finds itself once again in the midst of a global medical crisis. Throughout the state's history, its citizens have found themselves reminded, as they are reminded today, that they are connected with all the world's people via the pathogens that cause infectious disease. In the eighteenth century, the virus that causes yellow fever, along with the mosquito that transmitted the virus, emerged from West Africa, traversed the Atlantic, and changed the history of Philadelphia and the nation. In the nineteenth century, cholera, which hitherto spent thousands of years infecting only people adjacent to the Bay of Bengal, became for decades the most feared disease in the state, its very mention spurring communities to spring to action to avert calamity. The beginning of the twentieth century heralded a new era in medical science, in which the knowledge about the role of germs in infection was allied to new preventions and cures, such as clean water and various antitoxins. The optimism of this bold era was violently shaken when, in 1918, a virulent strain of influenza emerged, likely from rural southeastern China, and inflicted tens of thousands of deaths on the state. Pennsylvania's equanimity was again shattered in the 1980s, when HIV, a virus whose origins traced back almost a century to simian viruses that jumped from chimpanzees to people in equatorial Africa, leapt to our state and claimed thousands of victims.

Our commonwealth now faces a fresh challenge, a newly discovered coronavirus that moved in late 2019 from its natural reservoir in bats to the human population in China. In recent decades humanity has been lucky: though many lethal viruses responsible for diseases such as Marburg, Ebola, severe acute respiratory syndrome (SARS), Nipah, and Middle East respiratory syndrome (MERS) have emerged from bats, the spread of these pathogens, devastating as they might be for the people involved, has been limited to institutions or regions and never ignited a pandemic. The world's luck ended in January 2020, as COVID-19 spread well beyond China. By late February the virus was present in suburban Philadelphia, one of the first places in the United States to record cases of the disease. The parallels with the 1918 epidemic of influenza are stark: The governor and health department have activated emergency measures that closed most businesses and venues, and people accustomed to medicine's invincibility in the face of infection are left to contemplate not only the relative powerlessness of medicine against the new virus but also the necessity of relying on seemingly archaic public health responses, especially social distancing, which our ancestors termed simply "isolation." As individuals we meditate on the fact that our very bodies may be lethally dangerous to our loved ones, especially to the aged and those in poor health. Once again, as in 1918, schools and houses of worship stand empty, our main streets silent, our population largely sequestered behind closed doors.

Yet, as in 1918, our healthcare workers of every description risk their lives to save the sick while retired physicians and nurses, many of advanced age and highly susceptible to the disease, labor with little protection against the virus to rescue the lives of strangers. Funeral homes continue to offer dignity to the dead and their families, even if the number of people allowed to pay their respects in person is curtailed. Across Pennsylvania millions of people every day offer uncountable acts of kindness and love to their neighbors by providing a meal or simple words of encouragement.

As in our great commonwealth's past, its people give of themselves to lighten the burden of others during time of plague.

NOTES

Introduction

1. Allopathic medicine refers to mainstream, scientific medicine of the sort practiced by medical doctors, trained nurses, and hospitals. The term is most important in the context of conventional medicine as it developed during the nineteenth century and beyond.

Chapter 1

1. April M. Beisaw, "Environmental History of the Susquehanna Valley around the Time of European Contact," *Pennsylvania History: A Journal of Mid-Atlantic Studies* 79, no. 4 (Autumn 2012): 366–376.

2. Thomas J. Sugrue, "The Peopling and Depeopling of Early Pennsylvania: Indians and Colonists, 1680–1720," *Pennsylvania Magazine of History and Biography* 116, no. 1 (January 1992): 6–7.

3. The best work on the subject of the impact of disease on Native American populations is Alfred W. Crosby Jr., *The Columbian Exchange: Biological and Cultural Consequences of 1492* (Westport, CT: Greenwood, 1972).

4. George Henry Loskiel, *History of the Mission of the United Brethren among the Indians in North America*, trans. Christian Ignatius Latrobe (London: Brethren's Society for the Furtherance of the Gospel, 1794), 88, 112–114.

5. Ibid., 108.

6. Laurel Thatcher Ulrich, *A Midwife's Tale: The Life of Martha Ballard, Based on Her Diary, 1785–1812* (New York: Alfred A. Knopf, 1990), 62.

7. Susan Klepp, *Revolutionary Conceptions: Women, Fertility, and Family Limitation in America, 1760–1820* (Chapel Hill: University of North Carolina Press, 2009), 193–194.

8. Ulrich, *A Midwife's Tale*, 40.

9. Ibid., 51–52, 62–63.

10. David W. Kriebel, *Powwowing among the Pennsylvania Dutch: A Traditional Medical Practice in the Modern World* (University Park: Pennsylvania State University Press, 2007), 14–15.

11. Ibid., 100.

12. "Heads of Households, Pennsylvania," in *First Census of the United States, 1790* (Washington, DC: Government Printing Office, 1907–1908), 33.

13. Will of Anna Maria Young, entered into Berks County, Pa., register of wills, March 13, 1813–November 20, 1819.

14. Klepp, *Revolutionary Conceptions*, 241.

15. Use of the term "witch" is problematic for a number of reasons, not the least of which are the many negative connotations that surround the term. However, period writings often refer to powwow practitioners as witches or witch doctors, especially by the late nineteenth and early twentieth centuries when scientific medicine began to offer increasingly effective explanations and cures for infectious disease.

16. I spent several hours with the owners of the property in July 2017 and several days during the summers of 2016 and 2017 exploring the woods and ridges of the Oley Hills.

17. Susan E. Klepp, "Demography in Early Philadelphia, 1690–1860," *Proceedings of the American Philosophical Society* 133, no. 2 (June 1989): 99.

18. Charles S. Olton, "Philadelphia's First Environmental Crisis," *Pennsylvania Magazine of History and Biography* 98, no. 1 (January 1974): 91.

19. Elizabeth A. Fenn, *Pox Americana: The Great Smallpox Epidemic of 1775–82* (New York: Hill and Wang, 2001), 82–83.

20. Richard H. Shryock, "A Century of Medical Progress in Philadelphia: 1750–1850," *Pennsylvania History: A Journal of Mid-Atlantic Studies* 8, no. 1 (January 1941): 8.

21. Suzanne M. Schultz and Arthur E. Crist Jr., "Colonial Conundrum: Divining the Diagnosis of a Mysterious Fever," *Pennsylvania History: A Journal of Mid-Atlantic Studies* 78, no. 3 (Summer 2011): 274–275.

22. Ibid., 277.

23. Benjamin Rush, "An Account of the Bilious Remitting Fever as It Appeared in Philadelphia in the Summer and Autumn of the Year 1780," *American Journal of Medicine* 11, no. 5 (November 1951): 546–550.

24. Noga Arikha, *Passions and Tempers: A History of the Humours* (New York: HarperCollins, 2007).

25. Shryock, "A Century of Medical Progress in Philadelphia," 11.

26. James Leonard, untitled notice, *Pennsylvania Gazette*, September 11, 1740, p. 3.

27. Shryock, "A Century of Medical Progress in Philadelphia," 19.

28. Frederick P. Henry, ed., *Standard History of the Medical Profession of Philadelphia* (Chicago: Goodspeed Brothers, 1897), 37–38.

29. Shryock, "A Century of Medical Progress in Philadelphia," 12, 18.

30. Fenn, *Pox Americana*, 42.

31. John Redman Coxe, *Practical Observation on Vaccination: Or Inoculation for the Cow-Pock* (Philadelphia: James Humphreys, 1802), 46.

32. Klepp, *Revolutionary Conceptions*, 61.

33. Ibid., 281.

34. Elizabeth Drinker, *The Diary of Elizabeth Drinker: The Life Cycle of an Eighteenth-Century Woman*, abridged ed., ed. Elaine Forman Crane (Philadelphia: University of Pennsylvania Press, 2010), 147.

35. Henry, *Standard History of the Medical Profession of Philadelphia*, 41–45.

36. Sarah Blank Dine, "Diaries and Doctors: Elizabeth Drinker and Philadelphia Medical Practice, 1760–1810," *Pennsylvania History* 68, no. 4 (2001): 428.

37. Billy G. Smith, "Death and Life in a Colonial Immigrant City: A Demographic Analysis of Philadelphia," *Journal of Economic History* 37, no. 4 (December 1977): 879.

38. Klepp, *Revolutionary Conceptions*, 282–284.

39. Shryock, "A Century of Medical Progress in Philadelphia," 20.

40. Benjamin Rush, *Observations upon the Origins of the Malignant Bilious, or Yellow Fever in Philadelphia* (Philadelphia: Budd and Bartram, 1799), 9.

41. Henry, *Standard History of the Medical Profession of Philadelphia*, 23.

42. Thomas G. Morton, *The History of the Pennsylvania Hospital, 1751–1895* (Philadelphia: Times Printing House, 1897), 5.

43. Charles Lawrence, *History of the Philadelphia Almshouses and Hospitals* (Philadelphia: self-pub., 1905), 19, 20.

44. Morton, *History of the Pennsylvania Hospital*, 3, 4, 9.

45. William Pencak, "Free Health Care for the Poor: The Philadelphia Dispensary," *Pennsylvania Magazine of History and Biography* 136, no. 1 (January 2012): 25–52.

46. Henry, *Standard History of the Medical Profession of Philadelphia*, 106, 108.

47. Schultz and Crist, "Colonial Conundrum," 272–286.

48. Henry, *Standard History of the Medical Profession of Philadelphia*, 112.

49. Jacquelyn C. Miller, "The Wages of Blackness: African American Workers and the Meanings of Race during Philadelphia's 1793 Yellow Fever Epidemic," *Pennsylvania Magazine of History and Biography* 128, no. 2 (April 2005): 163–194.

50. Richard Allen and Absalom Jones, *A Narrative of the Proceedings of the Black People, during the Late Awful Calamity in Philadelphia in the Year 1793* (Philadelphia: William W. Woodward, 1794), 5.

51. Donald J. D'Elia, "Dr. Benjamin Rush and the Negro," *Journal of the History of Ideas* 30, no. 3 (July–September 1969): 415.

52. Henry, *Standard History of the Medical Profession of Philadelphia*, 109.

53. Rush, *Observations upon the Origins of the Malignant Bilious*, 9.

54. Henry, *Standard History of the Medical Profession of Philadelphia*, 117.

55. Ibid., 115.

56. Robert L. North, "Benjamin Rush, MD: Assassin or Beloved Healer?," *Proceedings of the Baylor University Medical Center* 13, no. 1 (January 2000): 45–49.

57. Henry, *Standard History of the Medical Profession of Philadelphia*, 118.

58. Ibid., 279, 288.

Chapter 2

1. Roger D. Simon, *Philadelphia: A Brief History* (Philadelphia: Pennsylvania Historical Association and Temple University Press, 2017), 38–39.

2. Philadelphia Medical Society, *Report of the Committee of the Medical Society of Philadelphia, on Epidemic Cholera* (Philadelphia: Lydia R. Bailey, 1832), 9–10.

3. John Duffy, "The Impact of Asiatic Cholera on Pittsburgh, Wheeling, and Charleston," *Western Pennsylvania Historical Magazine* 47, no. 3 (July 1964): 199–211.

4. William E. Watson, J. Francis Watson, John H. Ahtes III, and Earl H. Schandelmeier III, *The Ghosts of Duffy's Cut: The Irish Who Died Building America's Most Dangerous Stretch of Railroad* (Westport, CT: Praeger Press, 2006).

5. John B. Osborne, "The Lancaster County Cholera Epidemic of 1854 and the Challenge to the Miasma Theory of Disease," *Pennsylvania Magazine of History and Biography* 133, no. 1 (January 2009): 5–28.

6. Dora B. Weiner and Michael J. Sauter, "The City of Paris and the Rise of Clinical Medicine," *Osiris* 18 (2003): 23–42.

7. John Harley Warner, *Against the Spirit of System: The French Impulse in Nineteenth-Century American Medicine* (Baltimore: Johns Hopkins University Press, 1998), 32.

8. Richard H. Shryock, "A Century of Medical Progress in Philadelphia: 1750–1850," *Pennsylvania History: A Journal of Mid-Atlantic Studies* 8, no. 1 (January 1941): 23.

9. "Obituary," *Medical Times and Register* 2 (June 1872): 353.

10. William W. Gerhard, "On the Typhus Fever, Which Occurred at Philadelphia in the Spring and Summer of 1836," *American Journal of the Medical Sciences* (February 1837): 1–34.

11. Letter from Alfred Stille to George C. Shattuck, in Warner, *Against the Spirit of System*, 147.

12. Warner, *Against the Spirit of System*, 149.

13. Ibid., 257–260.

14. Walker Rumble, "Homeopathy in the Lehigh Valley, 1881–1920," *Pennsylvania Magazine of History and Biography* 104, no. 4 (October 1980): 475.

15. Shryock, "A Century of Medical Progress in Philadelphia," 26.

16. Marsha J. Hamilton, "Mercury and Water: Two Civil War Surgeons of the 148th Pennsylvania Volunteers," *Pennsylvania History: A Journal of Mid-Atlantic Studies* 75, no. 4 (Autumn 2008): 474.

17. Robert Rau and Elizabeth L. Meyers, "The Physicians of Early Bethlehem," *Transactions of the Moravians Historical Society* 11, no. 1 (1931): 56–61.

18. David W. Kriebel, *Powwowing among the Pennsylvania Dutch: A Traditional Medical Practice in the Modern World* (University Park: Pennsylvania State University Press, 2007), 101.

19. Charles E. Rosenberg, *The Care of Strangers: The Rise of America's Hospital System* (New York: Basic Books, 1987), 20–21.

20. Joanne Marie Andoirio, *Pillar of Pittsburgh: The History of Mercy Hospital and the City It Serves* (Pittsburgh, PA: Mercy Hospital, 1989).

21. Sarah Hutchins Killkelly, *The City of Pittsburgh: Its Rise and Progress* (Pittsburgh, PA: B. C. and Gordon Montgomery, 1906), 403.

22. Ibid., 386–389.

23. Elizabeth Blackwell, *Pioneer Work in Opening the Medical Profession to Women* (New York: Longmans, Green, 1895), 80.

24. Ibid., 80–81.

25. Ibid., 79.

26. Ibid.

27. Ibid., 81.

28. Shryock, "A Century of Medical Progress in Philadelphia," 26.

29. George W. Corner, *Two Centuries of Medicine: A History of the School of Medicine University of Pennsylvania* (Philadelphia: J. B. Lippincott, 1965), 108–109.

30. Frances Emily White, "The American Medical Woman," *Medical News* 67 (August 1895): 127.

31. Marie Lindhorst, "Politics in a Box: Sarah Mapps Douglass and the Female Literary Association, 1831–1833," *Pennsylvania History: A Journal of Mid-Atlantic Studies* 65, no. 3 (Summer 1998): 263–278.

32. U.S. National Library of Medicine, "Dr. Rebecca J. Cole," June 3, 2015, https://cfmedicine.nlm.nih.gov/physicians/biography_66.html.

33. White, "American Medical Woman," 126.

34. Warner, *Against the Spirit of System*, 233.

35. Howard Kistler Petry, ed., *A Century of Medicine, 1848–1948: The History of the Medical Society of the State of Pennsylvania* (Philadelphia: Medical Society of the State of Pennsylvania, 1952), 4–5.

36. Ibid., 34–35.

37. Ibid., 22–23, 35.

38. Shryock, "A Century of Medical Progress in Philadelphia," 21.

39. Charles Rosenberg, "What Is an Epidemic? AIDS in Historical Perspective," *Daedalus* 118, no. 2 (Spring 1989): 2.

40. J. M. Da Costa, "Biographical Sketch of Professor Samuel D. Gross," *Proceedings of the American Philosophical Society* 22, no. 117 (January 1885): 78.

41. Bennett A. Clements, "Memoir of Jonathan Letterman, M.D.," *Journal of the Military Service Institution* 4, no. 15 (1883): 1.

42. Ibid., 9.

43. Ibid., 10.

44. Winnifred K. MacKay, "Philadelphia during the Civil War, 1861–1865," *Pennsylvania Magazine of History and Biography* 70, no. 1 (January 1947): 28, 30.

45. Roberta Mayhew West, *History of Nursing in Pennsylvania* (Harrisburg, PA: Evangelical Press, 1939), 17–18.

46. Richard H. Shryock, "A Medical Perspective on the Civil War," *American Quarterly* 14, no. 2 (Summer 1962): 162.

47. Hamilton, "Mercury and Water," 476–477.

48. Robert L. Bloom, "'We Never Expected a Battle': The Civilians at Gettysburg, 1863," *Pennsylvania History: A Journal of Mid-Atlantic Studies* 55, no. 4 (October 1988): 181.

49. Ibid., 181.

50. Ibid., 179.

51. West, *History of Nursing in Pennsylvania*, 16–17.

52. Shryock, "A Century of Medical Progress in Philadelphia," 25.

53. Ibid., 25–26.

Chapter 3

1. B. Franklin Royer, "Doctor Dixon's Work in Sanitary Science," *Proceedings of the Academy of Natural Sciences of Philadelphia* 70, no. 1 (January–April 1918): 127.

2. George W. Corner, *Two Centuries of Medicine: A History of the School of Medicine University of Pennsylvania* (Philadelphia: J. B. Lippincott, 1965), 166, 181–182.

3. Earl H. Harley, "The Forgotten History of Defunct Black Medical Schools in the 19th and 20th Centuries and the Impact of the Flexner Report," *Journal of the National Medical Association* 98, no. 9 (September 2006): 1426. Nearby Cheyney University also lays claim to being the first black university because its roots as an educational institution stretch back to 1837, before it was a university.

4. Alfred Gordon, "Frederick Douglass Memorial Hospital and Training School," in *Philadelphia—World's Medical Centre,* edited by James M. Anders (Philadelphia: n.p., 1930), 58–59.

5. Ibid., 59.

6. Samuel G. Dixon, "Possibility of Establishing Tolerance for the Tubercle Bacillus," *Medical News* 55 (October 1889): 435.

7. Samuel G. Dixon, "Establishing Tolerance for the Tubercle Bacillus," *Medical and Surgical Reporter* 63 (September 1890): 281–282.

8. Walker Rumble, "Homeopathy in the Lehigh Valley, 1881–1920," *Pennsylvania Magazine of History and Biography* 104, no. 4 (October 1980): 474.

9. Owen Davies, *America Bewitched: The Story of Witchcraft after Salem* (Oxford: Oxford University Press, 2013), 149–150.

10. "Powwow Doctor Arrested," *Allentown Democrat,* October 17, 1894, p. 2.

11. "Convicted at Easton," *Allentown Democrat,* December 10, 1890, p. 3.

12. Karol Weaver, *Medical Caregiving and Identity in Pennsylvania's Anthracite Region, 1880–2000* (University Park: Pennsylvania State University Press, 2011), 86.

13. Ibid., 73.

14. *Pittsburgh's Fortresses of Health: 200 Years of Hospital Progress, 1758–1958* (Pittsburgh, PA: City of Pittsburgh, 1959), 6–18.

15. Edward T. Devine, "Results of the Pittsburgh Survey," *American Journal of Sociology* 14, no. 5 (March 1909): 661–662.

16. Abraham Epstein, *The Negro Migrant in Pittsburgh* (Pittsburgh, PA: University of Pittsburgh Press, 1918), 17.

17. Joel A. Tarr, ed., *Devastation and Renewal: An Environmental History of Pittsburgh and Its Region* (Pittsburgh, PA: University of Pittsburgh Press, 2003), 119.

18. Thomas Patrick Vadasz, "The History of an Industrial Community" (Ph.D. diss., College of William and Mary, 1975), 125.

19. Gordon B. Fister, *Half-Century: The Fifty-Year Story of the Allentown Hospital, 1899–1949* (Allentown, PA: H. Ray Haas, 1949).

20. Roberta Mayhew West, *History of Nursing in Pennsylvania* (Harrisburg, PA: Evangelical Press, 1939), 13–14.

21. West, *History of Nursing in Pennsylvania,* 734–736.

22. "In Memoriam S. Lillian Clayton, 1874–1930," *American Journal of Nursing* 30, no. 6 (June 1930): 686.

23. Roberta Mayhew West's exhaustive *History of Nursing in Pennsylvania* is the best source for reviewing the effects of hospital and nursing care in rural Pennsylvania as well as the character and impact of those schools on their communities.

24. West, *History of Nursing in Pennsylvania,* 105–107, 124–125.

25. Frederick P. Henry, ed., *Standard History of the Medical Profession of Philadelphia* (Chicago: Goodspeed Brothers, 1897), 290, 292.

26. Ibid., 297.

27. Jacqueline Karnell Corn, *Environment and Health in Nineteenth Century America: Two Case Studies* (New York: Peter Lang, 1989), 180.

28. Lincoln Steffens, *The Shame of the Cities* (New York: McClure, Philips, 1903), 160–164; "Boss Rule in Pennsylvania," *New York Times*, March 31, 1896, p. 4.

29. B. W. Kunkel, *Milestones to Health in Pennsylvania: A History of Public Health Work in the State* (self-pub., 1967), 41.

30. Benjamin Lee, "Sanitary Legislation in the Light of History: A Plea for a State Board of Health," *Penn Monthly* 9 (June 1878): 417–430.

31. Editorial, *Norristown Herald*, March 30, 1874, reprinted in "Paragraphs," *Harrisburg Telegraph*, March 31, 1974, p. 2.

32. Untitled news items column, *Harrisburg Telegraph*, March 11, 1881, p. 2.

33. "The Proposed Board of Health," *Harrisburg Telegraph*, February 25, 1875, p. 2; "Legislature," *Harrisburg Telegraph*, February 14, 1883, p. 1.

34. Benjamin Lee, "The Address in Hygiene," *Transactions of the Medical Society of the State of Pennsylvania at Its Twenty-Seventh Annual Session* 11, no. 1 (May–June 1876): 118.

35. In 2017 and 2019 the author climbed the length of Coal Creek. The water company breached the dams in the 1980s with the result that Coal Creek runs, much as it did before the 1870s, through an area of dense undergrowth within a steep-sided ravine. While the dams remain, and sections of cast-iron pipe are visible where water has eroded the ground, the holding ponds are now recognizable only as level areas in an otherwise steep slope. Near the fourth pond are the remains of the Davises' house, which lay near the traces of a road. Conditions mean access is limited to those with experience in traversing deep undergrowth without benefit of trail, markers, or signs.

36. Pennsylvania Board of Health and Vital Statistics, *Second Annual Report of the State Board of Health and Vital Statistics of the Commonwealth of Pennsylvania* (Harrisburg, PA: E. K. Meyers, 1886), 818–819.

37. Samuel G. Dixon and B. Franklin Royer, "Organization of the Pennsylvania State Department of Health," *Journal of the American Public Health Association* 36 (1911): 107.

38. Howard Kistler Petry, ed., *A Century of Medicine, 1848–1948: The History of the Medical Society of the State of Pennsylvania* (Philadelphia: Medical Society of the State of Pennsylvania, 1952), 99.

39. Josiah Granvil Leach, *History of the Penrose Family of Philadelphia* (Philadelphia: D. Biddle, 1903), 122.

40. John F. Anderson, "The Differentiation of Typhoid Fever due to Infection by Water, Milk, Flies, and Contact," *Medical Record: A Weekly Journal of Medicine and Surgery* 75, no. 22 (November 1908): 911.

41. Dixon and Royer, "Organization of the Pennsylvania State Department of Health," 107–108.

42. Samuel Whitaker Pennypacker, *The Autobiography of a Pennsylvanian* (Philadelphia: John C. Winston, 1918), 380.

Chapter 4

1. "On Wild Hunt for Black Cats," *Philadelphia Inquirer*, July 28, 1902, p. 1.

2. Owen Davies, *America Bewitched: The Story of Witchcraft after Salem* (Oxford: Oxford University Press, 2013), 151–152.

3. "Powwow Delusion Not Insanity, Rules Death Trial Judge," *Reading Times*, January 9, 1929, pp. 1–2.

4. "Prayer for 'Hex' Murderers Offered at Victim's Burial," *Reading Times*, December 3, 1928, p. 1.

5. Ibid.

6. Ibid.

7. Owners of Marie Jung's homestead and property, interview by the author, July 31, 2017, Berks County, PA.

8. Marietta Borough Office staff member, telephone interview by the author, August 8, 2017.

9. Richard Cain, telephone interview by the author, August 17, 2017.

10. Abraham Flexner, *Medical Education in the United States and Canada: A Report to the Carnegie Foundation for the Advancement of Education* (New York: Carnegie Foundation, 1910), 292.

11. Ibid., 293–297.

12. Ibid., 297–298.

13. Barbara I. Paull, *A Century of Medical Excellence: The History of the University of Pittsburgh School of Medicine* (Pittsburgh, PA: University of Pittsburgh Press, 1989), 48–50.

14. Mark A. Suckow, Steven H. Weisbroth, and Craig L. Franklin, eds., *The Laboratory Rat* (London: Elsevier Academic Press, 2006), 3–14.

15. Gretchen A. Condran, "The Elusive Role of Scientific Medicine in Mortality Decline: Diphtheria in Nineteenth- and Early Twentieth-Century Philadelphia," *Journal of the History of Medicine and Allied Sciences* 63, no. 4 (October 2008): 501.

16. B. Franklin Royer, "The Antitoxin Treatment of Diphtheria, with a Plea for Rational Dosage in Treatment and Immunizing," *Therapeutic Gazette* 29, no. 4 (April 1905): 217–227.

17. David Riesman, "The Pneumonia Situation in Philadelphia," *Transactions of the College of Physicians of Philadelphia* 39 (1917): 186.

18. The best study of medical specialization in Philadelphia is James A. Schafer Jr., *The Business of Private Medical Practice: Doctors, Specialization, and Urban Change in Philadelphia, 1900–1940* (New Brunswick, NJ: Rutgers University Press, 2014).

19. B. W. Kunkel, *Milestones to Health in Pennsylvania: A History of Public Health Work in the State* (self-pub., 1967), 63, 66, 69–70.

20. Samuel G. Dixon, "Protecting Public Health in Pennsylvania," *Annals of the American Academy of Political and Social Sciences* 37, no. 2 (March 1911): 95–102.

21. Samuel G. Dixon and B. Franklin Royer, "Organization of the Pennsylvania State Department of Health," *Journal of the American Public Health Association* 36 (1911): 116.

22. B. Franklin Royer, "Doctor Dixon's Work in Sanitary Science," *Proceedings of the Academy of Natural Sciences of Philadelphia* 70, no. 1 (January–April 1918): 132, 135, 138.

23. Joel A. Tarr, ed., *Devastation and Renewal: An Environmental History of Pittsburgh and Its Region* (Pittsburgh, PA: University of Pittsburgh Press, 2003), 72.

24. Edward T. Devine, "Results of the Pittsburgh Survey," *American Journal of Sociology* 14, no. 5 (March 1909): 661–662; G. E. Harmon, "A Comparison of the Relative Healthfulness of Certain Cities in the United States Based upon the Study of Their Vital Statistics," *Publications of the American Statistical Association* 15, no. 114 (June 1916): 164.

25. Paull, *A Century of Medical Excellence*, 81.

26. Bureau of the Census, *Financial Statistics of Cities Having a Population of over 30,000: 1918* (Washington, DC: Government Printing Office, 1919); Alfred W. Crosby, *America's Forgotten Pandemic: The Influenza of 1918*, 2nd ed. (New York: Cambridge University Press, 2003), 70.

27. Bethlehem War Chest, September 26, 1918, entry, in *Minute Book, 10 April 1918–30 December 1919*, Records of the United Way of Northampton and Warren Counties, 1918–1982, Bethlehem Public Library, Bethlehem, PA.

28. Department of Public Health and Charities, *Annual Report for the Year Ending December 31, 1918* (Philadelphia: City of Philadelphia, 1919), 144.

29. Abraham Epstein, *The Negro Migrant in Pittsburgh* (Pittsburgh, PA: University of Pittsburgh Press, 1918), 67.

30. Ibid., 56–58.

31. United States Public Health Service, "Poliomyelitis (Infantile Paralysis): Prevalence and Geographic Distribution during 1916," *Public Health Reports* 32, no. 26 (June 29, 1917): 1017.

32. Theodore Weisenburg, "Poliomyelitis: A Study of the 1916 Epidemic with a Report of 717 Cases," American Neurological Association, 1918, Historical Medical Library of the College of Physicians of Philadelphia.

33. Robert C. Alberts, *Pitt: The Story of the University of Pittsburgh, 1787–1987* (Pittsburgh, PA: University of Pittsburgh Press, 1986), 70.

34. W.M.L. Coplin, *American Red Cross Base Hospital No. 38 in the World War* (Philadelphia: W.M.L. Coplin, 1923).

35. E. G. Persons, "History of Camp Crane, Allentown, Pennsylvania," Lehigh County Historical Society, Allentown, PA.

36. Roberta Mayhew West, *History of Nursing in Pennsylvania* (Harrisburg, PA: Evangelical Press, 1939), 55.

37. Ibid., 31.

38. Ellen S. More, "'A Certain Restless Ambition': Women Physicians and World War I," *American Quarterly* 41, no. 4 (December 1989): 636–660.

39. B. Franklin Royer, "Mosquito Eradication in Southeastern Pennsylvania," *American Journal of Public Health* 9, no. 5 (May 1919): 327–332.

40. Department of Public Health and Charities, *Annual Report for the Year Ending December 31, 1918*, 485.

41. John Dill Robertson, *A Report on the Epidemic of Influenza in Chicago Occurring during the Fall of 1918* (Chicago: Chicago Department of Health, 1919), 48.

42. Mark Osborne Humphries, "Paths of Infection: The First World War and the Origins of the 1918 Influenza Pandemic," *War in History* 21, no. 1 (January 2014): 55–81.

43. Zong-Mei Sheng, Daniel S. Chertow, Xavier Ambroggio, Sherman McCall, Ronald M. Przygodzki, Robert E. Cunningham, Olga A. Maximova, John C. Kash, David M. Morens, and Jeffery K. Taubenberger, "Autopsy Series of 68 Cases Dying before and during the 1918 Influenza Pandemic Peak," *Proceedings of the National Academy of Sciences of the United States of America* 108, no. 39 (September 2011): 16416–16421.

44. Secretary of the Navy, *Annual Report of the Secretary of the Navy, 1919* (Washington, DC: Government Printing Office, 1920), 2424–2425.

45. Official Log Book No. 4, City of Exeter, July 21, 1918, Maritime History Archive, Memorial University of Newfoundland, Canada.

46. Bureau of Naval Personnel, *Officers and Enlisted Men of the United States Navy Who Lost Their Lives during the World War, from April 6, 1917 to November 11, 1918* (Washington, DC: Government Printing Office, 1920), 612.

47. "Medical News: Pennsylvania," *Journal of the American Medical Association* 71, no. 17 (October 26, 1918): 1424.

48. Pennsylvania Department of Health, *Pennsylvania's Health* (Harrisburg, PA: Government Printer, 1932), 27.

49. John O'Hara, "The Doctor's Son," in *Great Short Stories by John O'Hara: Stories from the Doctor's Son and Other Stories and Files on Parade* (New York: Bantam Books, 1965), 2.

50. Francis Edward Tourscher, *The Work of the Sisters during the Epidemic of Influenza, October 1918* (Philadelphia: American Catholic Historical Society, 1919), 275. This work is a book-length set of oral history compiled within a year of the epidemic's end and is the best firsthand account of the epidemic in Philadelphia.

51. Kunkel, *Milestones to Health in Pennsylvania*, 81.

52. Tourscher, *Work of the Sisters*, 2.

53. "Rapid Spread of Influenza in Pittsburgh," *Pittsburgh Gazette Times*, October 10, 1918, p. 1.

54. Perhaps the best clinical study of the epidemic in the nation is University of Pittsburgh School of Medicine, *Studies on Epidemic Influenza Comprising Clinical and Laboratory Investigation* (Pittsburgh: University of Pittsburgh School of Medicine, 1919).

Chapter 5

1. David M. Oshinsky, *Polio: An American Story* (New York: Oxford University Press, 2005), 116.

2. Herman P. Miller, ed., *Smull's Legislative Handbook and Manual of the State of Pennsylvania, 1918* (Harrisburg, PA: J.L.L. Kuhn, 1918), 278h–278i.

3. B. W. Kunkel, *Milestones to Health in Pennsylvania: A History of Public Health Work in the State* (self-pub., 1967), 193.

4. Ibid., 186.

5. Ibid., 126.

6. Charles Hardy III, "Using the Environmental History of the Commonwealth to Enhance Pennsylvania and U.S. History Courses," *Pennsylvania History: A Journal of Mid-Atlantic Studies* 79, no. 4 (Autumn 2012): 484.

7. Clarence A. Mills, "The Donora Episode," *Science* 3 (January 1950): 67–68.

8. Oshinsky, *Polio*, 61–62.

9. Ibid., 107–108.

10. There was some controversy surrounding Salk. For instance, the Cutter Incident, in which ten children were killed and scores left with varying degrees of paralysis when a defective Salk vaccine was administered, tarnished Salk's reputation, though he had nothing to do with the production of the vaccine that caused the tragedy. Salk could also be testy, even nasty, to colleagues, though his personality traits must be weighed against the sickness and deaths his work prevented, especially in children.

11. Victor Hrehorovich, William W. Dyal, and William D. Schrack, "Influenza Epidemic in Pennsylvania," *Health Services Report* 87, no. 9 (November 1972): 839.

12. The best study of emerging infectious diseases is Laurie Garrett, *The Coming Plague: Newly Emerging Diseases in a World Out of Balance* (New York: Penguin Books, 1994).

13. Eileen A. Lynch, "The Flu," *Philadelphia Bulletin Magazine*, November 19, 1978.

14. Gwyneth Cravens and John S. Karr, "Tracking Down the Epidemic," *New York Times Magazine*, December 12, 1976, p. 19.

15. Sean D. Hamill, "Did Bias Skew the CDC's Pittsburgh VA Legionnaires' Reports?" *Pittsburgh Post-Gazette*, December 11, 2016, https://www.post-gazette.com/news/health/2016/12/12/Did-bias-skew-the-CDC-s-Pittsburgh-VA-Legionnaires-reports/stories/201612120003.

16. "Best Medical Schools: Research," *U.S. News and World Report*, 2019, https://www.usnews.com/best-graduate-schools/top-medical-schools/research-rankings.

17. "U.S. News Announces the 2016–2017 Best Children's Hospitals," *U.S. News and World Report*, June 21, 2016, https://www.usnews.com/info/blogs/press-room/articles/2016-06-21/us-news-announces-the-2016-2017-best-childrens-hospitals; Penn Medicine, "U.S. News' Best Hospitals 'Honor Roll,'" https://www.pennmedicine.org/about/providing-quality-care/us-news-best-hospitals (accessed March 9, 2020).

18. UPMC, "Thomas P. Detre, M.D., Academic Leader and Architect of UPMC, Dies at 86," October 9, 2010, https://www.upmc.com/media/news/thomas-p-detre-md-academic-leader-architect-upmc-dies-86.

19. Arthur S. Levine, Thomas P. Detre, Margaret C. McDonald, Loren H. Roth, George A. Huber, Mary G. Brignano, Sandra N. Danoff, David M. Farner, Jeffrey L. Masnick, and Jeffrey A. Romoff, "The Relationship between the University of Pittsburgh School of Medicine and the University of Pittsburgh Medical Center—a Profile in Synergy," *Journal of the Association of American Medical Colleges* 83, no. 9 (September 2008): 816.

20. Nick Falsone, "Ranking the Lehigh Valley's 21 Biggest Private Employers," *Lehigh Valley Live*, January 5, 2017, https://www.lehighvalleylive.com/news/index.ssf/2017/01/ranking_the_lehigh_valleys_21.html.

21. Henry J. Kaiser Family Foundation, "The Pennsylvania Health Care Landscape," April 25, 2016, https://www.kff.org/health-reform/fact-sheet/the-pennsylvania-health-care-landscape/.

22. Stephen G. Post, "Compassionate Medical Care Benefits Professionals, Patients, Students and the Bottom Line," *Psychology Today*, July 29, 2011, https://www.psychologytoday.com/us/blog/the-joy-giving/201107/compassionate-medical-care-benefits-professionals-patients-students-and-3.

INDEX

Aedes aegypti, 13–14
Albert Einstein Hospital, 50
Allentown Hospital, 52, 53
American Medical Association, 36
Antibiotics, 74, 85–86, 88–90, 95; and tuberculosis 89–90

Bacterial revolution, 44–46
Barnes, Albert C., 48
Blackwell, Elizabeth, 33–34
Bleeding, 15
Blockley Hospital, 33–34, 58. *See also* Philadelphia General Hospital nursing school
Butler typhoid epidemic, 65

Calomel, 16
Camp Crane, 78–79, 83
Catholic Hospital of Pittsburgh, 50
Childbirth, 18
Children's Hospital of Philadelphia, 32, 99
Children's Hospital of Pittsburgh, 51
Cholera, 25–29; in western Pennsylvania, 27–28
Civil War medicine, 38–41
Clayton, S. Lillian, 54–56
College of the Physicians of Philadelphia, 16, 30

Country doctors, 8
County health departments, 92
County medical societies, 36
COVID-19, 106–107

Dengue fever, 14
Detre, Thomas, 99–100
Diphtheria, 12–13, 39; antitoxin for, 46, 72–73
Dixon, Samuel G., 46–47, 48, 65–66, 74–76, 82
Donora smoke tragedy, 92

Eye and Ear Hospital of Pittsburgh, 51

Family care of sick, 7–8
Family planning, 19
Fisher, Alice, 54–56
Flexner Report, 72
Frederick Douglass Memorial Hospital and Training School, 47
Friends Almshouse, 20
Friends Hospital, 32

Gerhard, William W., 29–30
Gettysburg, Battle of, 40–41
Gross, Samuel D., 39

Hex murders, 69–71
HIV/AIDS, 97–99, 103
Homeopathy, 30–31, 34–35, 42–43, 49; Homeopathic Medical and Surgical Hospital and Dispensary, 50
Horner, Edith, 54, 56, 57
Hospital construction, 50–52
Hospital of the University of Pennsylvania, 50, 99

Influenza: 1918–1922 pandemic, 80–86; 1957–1958 pandemic, 95; 1968 pandemic, 95
Irish, as blamed for cholera, 26–28
Iron lung, 92–93

Jefferson Medical College, 32, 35, 47, 72
Jung, Anna Marie, 9–11, 71

Koch, Robert, 45–46
Krusen, Wilmer, 80, 81, 84–85

Labor and delivery, 18
Lancaster cholera outbreak, 28–29
Lee, Benjamin, 61, 63–64
Legionnaires' disease, 1, 96–97, 103
Lehigh Valley Health Network, 101
Letterman, Jonathan, 39–40
Lincoln University School of Medicine, 47
Lister, Joseph, 45

Malaria, 14, 39
Measles, 12–13, 39
Medical Society of Pennsylvania, 36–37, 61; negative effect of, on irregular healers, 36; negative effect of, on women physicians, 36
Mercury as treatment for disease, 16–17
Mercy Hospital, 33
Midwives, 8, 18–19, 52
Mossell, Nathan Francis, 47
Mountain Mary, 9–11, 71

Native Americans: contact of, with Europeans, 6–7; and disease, 6; European views of, 7; treatments of disease by, 6–7
Nursing, 52–57
Nursing Society of Philadelphia, 53

Opioid epidemic, 102
Opium, 17

Paris School of Medicine, 29–30
Passavant Hospital, 33
Pasteur, Louis, 45
Pennsylvania Board of Health, 60–65; resistance to, 61–62
Pennsylvania Department of Health, 65–66, 74–76, 90–91; and tuberculosis control and treatment, 75–76
Pennsylvania Dutch healing practices, 8–11, 105
Pennsylvania Hospital, 20–21; nursing school of, 54, 81
Penrose, Charles, 65
Philadelphia: board of health for, 23, 58–59; cholera in, 26–29; colonial, 11–12; endemic smallpox in, 13; influenza in, 81, 83–85; public health in, 19–20
Philadelphia Almshouse, 20
Philadelphia Dispensary, 21
Philadelphia General Hospital nursing school, 54–57
Phipps Institute, 73
Pittsburgh: air pollution in, 91; influenza in, 81, 84–85; public health in, 59–60, 77; typhoid in, 77
Plymouth typhoid epidemic, 62–63
Pneumonia, 73, 80
Polio, 4, 78, 92–94
Powwow, 9–10, 31–32, 34, 48–50, 69–71
Premodern disease explanations, 14–15

Quarantine of ships, 20

Regional health network, 100–101
Royer, B. Franklin, 72–73, 75, 80, 82–82, 85
Rural healers, 8, 11
Rush, Benjamin, 16, 21–22; and yellow fever controversy, 22–23

Salk, Jonas, 93–94
Scarlet fever, 12–13
Shippen, William, 16
Shippen, William, Jr., 16
Slaves as healers, 15–16

Smallpox, 12–13; inoculation of, 17–18, 34
Snow, John, 28–29
St. Francis Hospital of Pittsburgh, 50
St. Luke's Hospital, 52, 101; nursing school of, 54
Swine flu, 96–97, 103

Temple University School of Medicine, 47, 72
Tetanus, 46
Thomas Jefferson University Hospital, 32
Typhoid, 62–63, 65, 77

United States Sanitary Commission, 40; and sanitary fairs, 40
University of Pennsylvania School of Medicine, 16, 35, 46, 72, 99
University of Pittsburgh Medical Center, 100

University of Pittsburgh School of Medicine, 47, 72, 100

Water cure, 31, 34–35, 42–43, 49
Western Pennsylvania Hospital, 33
Western Pennsylvania Medical College, 47. *See also* University of Pittsburgh School of Medicine
Women's Medical College of Pennsylvania, 35–36, 52, 72; African American physicians at, 35–36
World War I: doctor shortage as a result of, 79–80; population during, 77–78

Yellow fever, 1, 12, 14, 21–23, 25; African American response to, 22

James E. Higgins is a lecturer in History at Rider University and researches the history of medicine in America and abroad. He is the winner of the 2015 Philip S. Klein Pennsylvania History Prize.